AF880875

Bodily Exchanges, Bioethics and Border Crossing

Medical therapy, research and technology enable us to make our bodies, or parts of them, available to others in an increasing number of ways. This is the case in organ, tissue, egg and sperm donation as well as in surrogate motherhood and clinical research. Bringing together leading scholars working on the ethical, social and cultural aspects of such bodily exchanges, this cutting-edge book develops new ways of understanding them.

Bodily Exchanges, Bioethics and Border Crossing both probes the established giving and selling frameworks for conceptualising bodily exchanges in medicine, and seeks to develop and examine another, less familiar framework: that of sharing. A framework of sharing can capture practices that involve giving up and giving away part of one's body, such as organ and tissue donation, and practices that do not, such as surrogacy and research participation. Sharing also recognizes the multiple relationalities that these exchanges can involve and invites inquiry into the context in which they occur. In addition, the book explores the multiple forms of border crossing that bodily exchanges in medicine involve, from the physical boundaries of the body to relational borders – as can happen in surrogacy – to national borders and the range of ethical issues that these various border crossings can give rise to.

Engaging with anthropology, sociology, philosophy, and feminist and postcolonial perspectives, this is an original and timely contribution to contemporary bioethics in a time of increasing globalization. It will be of use to students and researchers from a range of humanities and social science backgrounds as well as medical and other healthcare professionals with an interest in bioethics.

Erik Malmqvist, PhD, is Associate Professor in Medical Ethics at the Department of Thematic Studies: Technology and Social Change, Linköping University, Sweden. His research interests include ethical issues in organ and tissue transplantation, biomedical research, assisted reproduction and vaccination. Currently his research focuses on the ethics of international clinical research and of commodifying the human body. His publications have appeared in journals such as *The Lancet, Bioethics, Hastings Center Report, Journal of Medical Ethics* and *Journal of Applied Philosophy*.

Kristin Zeiler, PhD, is Professor at the Department of Thematic Studies: Technology and Social Change, Linköping University, Sweden, and *Pro Futura Scientia* Fellow at the Swedish Collegium for Advanced Study, Uppsala University, Sweden. Zeiler examines ethical, social and cultural aspects of biotechnological interventions and explores how medical treatment, the use of new technology and experience of pain and illness can form our ways of engaging with others and the world, and inform our self-understandings. Her research areas include medical humanities, bioethics, philosophy of medicine and feminist theory, and among her publications is the edited volume (with L.F. Käll) *Feminist Phenomenology and Medicine* (2014). Zeiler's articles have appeared in journals such as *Bioethics, Feminist Theory* and *Medicine, Health Care and Philosophy*.

Routledge Studies in the Sociology of Health and Illness

Available titles include:

Dimensions of Pain
Humanities and Social Science Perspectives
Edited by Lisa Folkmarson Käll

Aging Men, Masculinities and Modern Medicine
Edited by Antje Kampf, Barbara L. Marshall and Alan Petersen

Disclosure in Health and Illness
Mark Davis and Lenore Manderson

Caring and Well-being
A Lifeworld Approach
Kathleen Galvin and Les Todres

Systems Theory and the Sociology of Health and Illness
Observing Healthcare
Edited by Morten Knudsen and Werner Vogd

Complaints, Controversies and Grievances in Medicine
Edited by Jonathan Reinarz and Rebecca Wynter

The Public Shaping of Medical Research
Patient Associations, Health Movements and Biomedicine
Edited by Peter Wehling and Willy Viehöver

Giving Blood
The Institutional Making of Altruism
Edited by Johanne Charbonneau and André Smith

Health, Food and Social Inequality
Critical Perspectives on the Supply and Marketing of Food
Carolyn Mahoney

Gendered Violence, Abuse and Mental in Everyday Lives
Beyond Trauma
Nicole Moulding

Bodily Exchanges, Bioethics and Border Crossing
Perspectives on Giving, Selling and Sharing Bodies
Edited by Erik Malmqvist and Kristin Zeiler

Forthcoming titles:

Vaginal Examination in Labour
Challenging Contemporary Practice
Mary Stewart

Transnationalising Reproduction
Third Party Conception in a Globalised World
Edited by Roisin Ryan Flood and Jenny Gunnarsson Payne

The Social Determinants of Male Health
John MacDonald

Fathering Children with Autism
Needs, Practices and Service Use
Carol Potter

Bodily Exchanges, Bioethics and Border Crossing

Perspectives on giving, selling and sharing bodies

Edited by
Erik Malmqvist and Kristin Zeiler

Routledge
Taylor & Francis Group
LONDON AND NEW YORK

First published 2016
by Routledge
4 Park Square, Milton Park, Abingdon, Oxon OX14 4RN

and by Routledge
605 Third Avenue, New York, NY 10017

Routledge is an imprint of the Taylor & Francis Group, an informa business

© 2016 E. Malmqvist and K. Zeiler

The right of Erik Malmqvist and Kristin Zeiler to be identified as the authors of the editorial material, and of the authors for their individual chapters, has been asserted in accordance with sections 77 and 78 of the Copyright, Designs and Patents Act 1988.

All rights reserved. No part of this book may be reprinted or reproduced or utilised in any form or by any electronic, mechanical, or other means, now known or hereafter invented, including photocopying and recording, or in any information storage or retrieval system, without permission in writing from the publishers.

Trademark notice: Product or corporate names may be trademarks or registered trademarks, and are used only for identification and explanation without intent to infringe.

British Library Cataloguing in Publication Data
A catalogue record for this book is available from the British Library

Library of Congress Cataloging in Publication Data
Bodily exchanges, bioethics and border crossing : perspectives on giving, selling and sharing bodies / edited by Erik Malmqvist and Kristin Zeiler.
p. ; cm. -- (Routledge studies in the sociology of health and illness)
Includes bibliographical references and index.
I. Malmqvist, Erik, editor. II. Zeiler, Kristin, 1973- , editor. III. Series: Routledge studies in the sociology of health and illness.
[DNLM: 1. Tissue and Organ Procurement--ethics. 2. Transplantation--ethics. 3. Reproductive Techniques, Assisted--ethics. WO 690]
RA1063.3
174.2'97954--dc23
2015026424

ISBN: 978-1-138-85876-3 (hbk)
ISBN: 978-1-315-71776-0 (ebk)

Typeset in Times New Roman
by Taylor & Francis Books

Contents

Contributors

Simone Bateman, PhD, is a sociologist and Emeritus Senior Researcher of the French National Centre for Scientific Research (CNRS), working at the Centre for Research on Medicine, Science, Health and Society (CERMES3) in Paris, France. Most of her work focuses on morally controversial medical and scientific practices, primarily in the area of reproduction, and on bioethics as a historically specific social phenomenon. She has contributed to reports for French and European institutions, notably a European Commission report on reproductive technology, *Fertility and the Family* (1989). She has been a member of the French National Ethics Committee from 1992 to 1996 and has recently co-edited two volumes on enhancement (with J. Gayon, S. Allouche, J. Goffette and M. Marzano): *Inquiring into Human Enhancement: Interdisciplinary and International Perspectives* (2015) and *Inquiring into Animal Enhancement: Model or Countermodel of Human Enhancement?* (2015).

Leonardo D. de Castro, PhD, is Professor and Senior Research Fellow at the Centre for Biomedical Ethics, Yong Loo Lin School of Medicine, National University of Singapore. His main research interests are in the area of organ transplantation ethics, research ethics, genetic and genomic research ethics, bioethics education and Filipino philosophy. De Castro has published books in the Filipino language, one of which won him a National Book Award in 1998. He is Editor-in-Chief at *Asian Bioethics Review*, serves on the editorial advisory board of around 10 other international journals, and has been Vice Chair of the UNESCO International Bioethics Committee, Secretary of the International Association of Bioethics and Vice Chair of the Asian Bioethics Association.

Erica Haimes, PhD, FAcSS, is Professor of Sociology and the Founding Executive Director of the PEALS (Policy, Ethics and Life Sciences) Research Centre, at Newcastle University, UK. Her research interests include interdisciplinary research on social, ethical and legal aspects of the life sciences, reproductive and genetic technologies, socio-ethical aspects of the provision of human tissue for research, and the relationship between states, families and medicine with a focus on assisted conception. Haimes founded the PARTS (Provision and Acquisition of Reproductive Tissue for Science) International Research Network, and has been a member of various policy and practice ethics advisory bodies including for UK Biobank, the International Society for Stem Cell Research and the UK's Royal College of Obstetrics and Gynaecology. She is a full council member on the UK's Nuffield Council on Bioethics.

Michael Humbracht is a PhD candidate in Tourism and Hospitality Management at the University of Surrey, UK. He researches within mobility studies, focused specifically on intersections of tourism and migration. Humbracht's PhD is on Italian migrant practices of keeping touch with friends and family in Italy, and his recent publications include "Reimagining transnational relations: the embodied politics of visiting friends and relatives mobilities", *Population, Space and Place* (2015) and "Making palpable connections: objects in migrants transnational lives", *Ethnologia Scandinavica* (2013).

Insoo Hyun, PhD, is Associate Professor of Bioethics and Philosophy at Case Western Reserve University School of Medicine, USA. His research interests include ethical and policy issues in stem cell research, research ethics and informed consent, and medical decision-making. Hyun has published extensively and his bioethics articles have appeared in *Science, Nature, Cell Stem Cell, The Hastings Center Report* and *The Kennedy Institute of Ethics Journal*, as some examples. Recently, he has also published the book *Bioethics and the Future of Stem Cell Research* (2013).

Susanne Lundin, PhD, is Professor of Ethnology at the Department of Arts and Cultural Sciences, Lund University, Sweden, and Fellow at the Stellenbosch Institute for Advanced Study (STIAS), South Africa. Her main research area is cultural analysis of medical praxis. Her research on medical travel has been published in various articles and books, most recently, in the book *Organs for Sale: An Ethnographic Examination of the International Organ Trade* (2015).

Erik Malmqvist, PhD, is Associate Professor in Medical Ethics at the Department of Thematic Studies: Technology and Social Change, Linköping University, Sweden. His research interests include ethical issues in organ and tissue transplantation, biomedical research, assisted reproduction and vaccination. Currently his research focuses on the ethics of international clinical research and of commodifying the human body. Malmqvist's publications have appeared in journals such as *The Lancet, Bioethics, Hastings Center Report, Journal of Medical Ethics* and *Journal of Applied Philosophy.*

Donna McCormack, PhD, is a Research Fellow at the Centre for Women's and Gender Research (SKOK) at the University of Bergen, Norway. Her main research interests are biotechnologies in fiction, evolutionary theory, postcolonial studies and queer theory. Her current project focuses on the representation of organ transplantation in contemporary postcolonial literary and cinematic texts. Among her recent publications are the book *Queer Postcolonial Narratives and the Ethics of Witnessing* (2014), and the articles "Transplant temporalities and deadly reproductive futurity in Alejandro González Iñárritu's *21 Grams*", *European Journal of Cultural Studies* (2015), and "The ethics of biomedical tourism" and "Hopeful monsters: a queer hope for evolutionary difference", both in *Somatechnics* (2015).

Joseph Millum, PhD, holds a joint faculty appointment with the Clinical Center Department of Bioethics and the Fogarty International Center at the National Institutes of Health, Bethesda, USA. His current research focuses on the rights and responsibilities of parents, global justice and bioethics, priority setting for global health and international research ethics. He is co-editor of the book *Global Justice and Bioethics* (2012).

Lesley A. Sharp, PhD, is a medical anthropologist and Ann Whitney Olin Professor in Anthropology at Barnard College and Senior Research Scientist in Sociomedical Sciences at the Mailman School of Public Health, Columbia University, USA. Her research concerns include indigenous healing in Madagascar, human organ transfer in the USA and, most recently, the socio-moral consequences of highly experimental transplant science in five Anglophone countries. Sharp is the author of the book *Strange Harvest: Organ Transplants, Denatured Bodies, and the Transformed Self*, which won the New Millennium Book Award from the Society for Medical Anthropology; *The Transplant Imaginary: Mechanical Hearts, Animal Parts, and Moral Thinking in Highly Experimental Science*; and co-editor (with N. Chen) of *Bioinsecurity and Vulnerability*. She is currently working on a book addressing the everyday ethics in branches of laboratory science that employ animals as experimental subjects.

Fredrik Svenaeus, PhD, is Professor at the Centre for Studies in Practical Knowledge, Södertörn University, Sweden. His main research areas are philosophy of medicine, bioethics, medical humanities and philosophical anthropology. Current research projects focus on the concept of suffering in bioethics and on psychiatric diagnosis and the concept of medicalization. Recent publications include: "The phenomenology of suffering in medicine and bioethics", *Theoretical Medicine and Bioethics* (2014), "Organ transplantation ethics from the perspective of embodied selfhood", *The Routledge Companion to Bioethics* (2015) and "The relationship between empathy and sympathy in good health care", *Medicine, Health Care and Philosophy* (2015).

Sarah Jane Toledano is a PhD candidate in Health and Society at the Department of Thematic Studies: Technology and Social Change, Linköping University, Sweden. Her PhD project is a combined empirical and philosophical study of altruistic surrogate motherhood between families and friends. Her research interests include: bioethical issues of commodification and exploitation within developing countries; ethics and relationality in assisted reproductive technologies; and feminist phenomenological approaches.

Kristin Zeiler, PhD, is Professor at the Department of Thematic Studies: Technology and Social Change, Linköping University, Sweden, and *Pro Futura Scientia* Fellow at the Swedish Collegium for Advanced Study, Uppsala University, Sweden. Zeiler examines ethical, social and cultural aspects of biotechnological interventions and explores how medical treatment, the use of new technology and experience of pain and illness can form our ways of engaging with others and the world, and inform our self-understandings. Her research areas include medical humanities, bioethics, philosophy of medicine and feminist theory, and among her publications is the edited volume (with L.F. Käll) *Feminist Phenomenology and Medicine* (2014). Zeiler's articles have appeared in journals such as *Bioethics, Feminist Theory* and *Medicine, Health Care and Philosophy.*

1 Introduction

Bodily exchanges, bioethics and border crossing

Kristin Zeiler and Erik Malmqvist

Bodily exchanges in medicine

Medical practice and research increasingly involve making individuals' bodies, or parts of them, available to others in different ways. The paradigmatic example is organ transplantation. Since its inception as a highly experimental treatment in the 1950s, kidney transplantation has become increasingly commonplace, with at least 77,800 transplants performed worldwide in 2012 according to the WHO.[1] A key step in this development was the discovery of cyclosporine in the 1970s, which made it possible to suppress the body's immune system and drastically reduce the rejection problems that afflicted transplantation in its early days. With this drug available, transplant surgeons soon turned to other organs. Today the whole or parts of the heart, lungs, liver, pancreas, intestine and thymus are also transplanted (some on an experimental basis) from living or deceased donors into the bodies of ailing recipients.

In addition to organs, a number of bodily tissues and cell types are transferred between bodies for therapeutic purposes. Blood transfusions and skin allografts have formed part of routine clinical practice for many decades, and both have a pre-history stretching much further back.[2] Corneas, heart valves, bones and tendons, most often procured from deceased donors, are also transplanted on a large scale. Moreover, a source of therapies for patients with leukaemia and a few other diseases are stem cells harvested from living donors' bone marrow or blood, or in some cases from umbilical cord blood obtained at a child's birth.

In all these cases, organs and tissues are transferred for the sake of somebody else's survival or health. However, a person's bodily material can also be used to serve other people's reproductive interests or to advance biomedical research. Donated sperm, eggs and embryos are used in assisted reproduction to overcome different forms of infertility, and recently the first child gestated in a transplanted uterus was born (Brännström *et al.* 2015). Because of how assisted reproduction attempts are performed, they typically yield more fertilized eggs than are needed for implantation in the prospective mother's uterus. These "surplus" embryos constitute a prized resource for human embryonic stem cell research, an experimental scientific field often claimed to harbour great therapeutic potential. Further, some tissues commonly discarded as waste in clinical practice – in particular certain cancer tissues – have proven highly exploitable for scientific and commercial ends.

Other biomedical practices involve not the transfer of discrete body parts, but rather the temporary use of individuals' entire bodies for the benefit of others. For instance, the development of new drugs and other medical interventions requires extensive testing on large numbers of human subjects in randomized controlled trials. Another example is gestational surrogacy, where a woman agrees to become pregnant through in vitro fertilization and relinquish the child to the intended parents after delivery.

This volume examines a wide range of ways in which people's bodies or body parts are made available to others in medicine.[3] We will refer to all these uses of bodies as *bodily exchanges*. Our use of this term is deliberately inclusive, encompassing not only literal transfers where one party gives up something that another receives (e.g. organ transplantation) but also the accessing and altering of some individuals' bodies in order to benefit others (e.g. clinical research).[4] Though diverging somewhat from ordinary language, this inclusiveness has an analytic point. By drawing together a set of practices that appear highly diverse and that have mostly been analysed separately in previous research, but that nonetheless share important features, we seek to render visible unexamined similarities and differences.

In keeping with this inclusive approach, the volume contains contributions from authors working in a range of different areas of scholarly inquiry: anthropology, ethnology, sociology, postcolonial and feminist studies, bioethics, and continental as well as analytic philosophy. We find this diversity of perspectives quite fitting in view of the subject matter that is being addressed. Bodily exchanges in medicine are differentiated, multifaceted and constantly changing phenomena, lending themselves to many different styles of analysis and argument.

An organizing theme for the different chapters of this volume is the *boundary-crossing* nature of bodily exchanges in medicine. Not only do these exchanges transcend the body's physical limits in different ways, but this obvious form of boundary-crossing is commonly bound up with a less obvious one: the crossing and redrawing of *relational boundaries*. For instance, surrogate mothers in intrafamilial or friend-to-friend arrangements narrate how they form deep bonds with intending mothers during pregnancy while simultaneously restricting their engagement with their own partners (Toledano and Zeiler 2016). Similarly, organ donation can engender surprisingly intense connections between donors or their kin and recipients, despite transplant professionals' insistence on anonymity (Sharp 2006). This dual capacity of bodily exchanges to bridge and create divides between people is addressed by several of the contributors to this volume.

Bodily exchanges in medicine also tend to approach, stretch or transgress the *limits of the socially accepted* in different ways and to different degrees.

The exchanges analysed in this volume are, or have at least at some point been, perceived to raise ethical concern, and are in consequence surrounded by extensive scholarly and public debate as well as governed by elaborate legal and regulatory frameworks. The ethical, social, and cultural complexities of these exchanges are at the forefront of the authors' analyses.

Moreover, bodily exchanges increasingly cross *national* borders. A dramatic example is the illegal global kidney trade, which connects renal patients from affluent countries with kidney vendors from low-income countries (Scheper-Hughes 2003; Shimazono 2007; Lundin 2015). Other controversial practices are transnational commercial surrogacy arrangements, where women in India, for instance, are paid to carry and give birth to a child for infertile foreign couples (Pande 2009, 2010; Vora 2013), and the growing "offshoring" of clinical trials to emerging economies in Eastern Europe, Asia and Latin America (Petryna 2009; Cooper and Waldby 2014). Furthermore, human cells and tissues intended for transplantation, reproduction and research are increasingly circulated in complex global exchange systems involving both commercial and non-commercial agents (Waldby and Mitchell 2006; Schulz-Baldes *et al.* 2007; Whittaker and Speier 2010; Inhorn 2011; Nahman 2012).

The transnational dimension adds further layers to the ethical, social and cultural complexities surrounding bodily exchanges in medicine, and scholars are still struggling to make sense of the new situation. There is thus an important challenge here, which this volume seeks to take up. The increasingly transnational nature of bodily exchanges is a recurrent topic in the chapters that will follow.

In addition to highlighting the boundary-crossing nature of bodily exchanges in medicine, the volume seeks to contribute to scholarly debates about them in a further way. It explores the implications of conceptualizing these exchanges not as a transfer of gifts or commodities, as they are typically understood, but instead as an act of sharing. In the remainder of this chapter we explain the rationale for this shift in perspective, and in the concluding chapter we explore its implications more extensively.

Two ethical frameworks

As pointed out above, bodily exchanges in medicine are to varying degrees considered ethically controversial. Consequently, healthcare professionals, policy makers and scholars have spent considerable time and energy seeking to specify how individuals should engage in these exchanges and how institutions should regulate and incentivize them. Two ethical frameworks guide contemporary thinking about these issues. The reigning framework has long been that of *gift giving*. In this framework, exchanged body parts and bodily services are understood as gifts, and those who provide them are typically conceptualized as engaging in a generous and caring act. The exchange is framed as being performed voluntarily, for the benefit of others and without any expectation of personal gain (except, perhaps, the "gain" of knowing that one contributes to somebody else's health or happiness).[5]

The website of a hospital in Malmö, Sweden, provides a striking illustration of this framework. Along with information about egg donation, including what to do if one wants to become a donor, the website displays a picture of a chicken egg wrapped in red strings of the sort typical for birthday presents. The viewer is asked: would you like to give something really, really valuable?[6] In a similar vein, public campaigns aimed at encouraging organ donation often draw on a gift-of-life discourse, which sets the gift of an organ apart from other gifts as an especially valuable, or indeed *invaluable*, gift of life (Joralemon 1995; Siminoff and Chillag 1999).

Empirical studies show that features of the gift-giving framework figure in donors', recipients' and healthcare professionals' views on organ donation (Sque *et al.* 2007; Shaw 2010). For instance, the notion of the gift is invoked by transplant coordinators in order to emphasize that donation should be selfless and non-reciprocal, i.e. that "there are no strings attached" (Shaw 2010, 613). Moreover, the framework is widely invoked in national and international laws, regulations and guidelines, typically as an antithesis to commercial bodily exchanges, which are prohibited or severely circumscribed in most countries. For instance, the Declaration of Istanbul, whose condemnation of organ trafficking and transplant tourism has been endorsed by medical and transplantation societies worldwide and has influenced legislation in many countries, urges that transplantation be considered "the gift of health by one individual to another" (Participants in the International Summit on Transplant Tourism and Organ Trafficking 2008, 854).

While the gift framework is widely endorsed, it comes in different versions, and different rationales have been provided in its support. Some primarily appear to consider gift giving a praiseworthy individual act that reflects the provider's generous intention or disposition.[7] For others, it is a valuable social practice that expresses and contributes to societal cohesion and solidarity among citizens (Titmuss 1970; Murray 1987; Chambers 2001). Though analytically distinct, these rationales are not uncommonly invoked together and in support of each other (Joralemon 1995). Yet another rationale for the gift framework is the idea that it is appropriate that we give what we no longer need because we have ourselves been given our bodily existence by others (Svenaeus 2010).

The gift framework has been criticized for hiding or downplaying the darker sides of bodily exchanges in medicine. Surrogacy, research participation and most forms of living organ, tissue and cell donation involve physical risks and inconveniences of varying kinds and magnitudes. Moreover, in the transplantation context, scholars have argued that donation is often emotionally difficult, and that it can be the result of social pressures and power dynamics (Fox and Swazey 2002; Scheper-Hughes 2007). Such potentially problematic aspects arguably disappear from view when body parts or bodily services are understood as freely and voluntarily given.

A different concern is that the gift framework encourages feelings of indebtedness and counter-gifts on the part of recipients. Drawing on Marcel

Mauss' (1967 [1923–1924]) analysis of the threefold obligations to give, receive and reciprocate governing gift exchanges in archaic societies, scholars have emphasized that organ donation can involve an implicit expectation of reciprocity that may be difficult or even impossible for recipients to fulfil, engendering what has been called "the tyranny of the gift" (Fox and Swazey 2002, 40; Scheper-Hughes 2007). The widespread gift rhetoric surrounding transplantation has been criticized for reinforcing such experiences and for enabling healthcare professionals to use these experiences to manipulate recipients' behaviour in desired ways (Siminoff and Chillag 1999).

Yet another critique of the gift framework is that it is hypocritical and perhaps unfair (Mahoney 2000; Erin and Harris 2003). Providers of body parts and bodily services are vigorously encouraged to give without expecting anything in return, while the other parties involved in the exchange – recipients, medical personnel, and in some cases researchers and biotech and pharmaceutical companies – all derive significant, and often financial, gain.

Moreover, the gift framework requires specifying when the involvement of money is compatible with giving and when it turns exchanges into sales – a distinction that has proved elusive. While the gift framework proscribes outright commerce, in practice it coexists with various forms of financial transfer that are considered acceptable: reimbursement of costs incurred as a result of donating, including lost income, and sometimes compensation for risks and inconveniencies (WHO 2010, 5; Pennings *et al.* 2014; Krolokke 2014). In principle these transfers differ from purchases in that they seek to remove obstacles for those who are already inclined to donate for altruistic reasons rather than incentivizing those who lack altruistic motivation. But this distinction is less neat in practice: payment intended as reimbursement or compensation under a gift framework sometimes results in the recruitment of financially motivated providers (Cooper and Waldby 2014; Pennings *et al.* 2014). This is not surprising. A given sum may barely offset the burdens of donation for one person while constituting a positive incentive for another, depending on differences in, for example, financial situation, tolerance for risk and discomfort, and available options for raising income and providing for one's family. Thus, as long as the gift framework permits *some* form of financial transfer to providers, it arguably opens the door for precisely the sort of commercial exchanges that it seeks to rule out.

In response to perceived difficulties with the gift framework, many commentators have instead advocated a framework of *selling*. Proponents of this framework hold that bodily exchanges (or some such exchanges) should be considered market exchanges in decisive respects and that the exchanged body parts or services should be considered commodities. Though its influence on policy and practice is limited, such a framework does govern bodily exchanges in certain geographical and medical areas. In many states in the USA gametes are procured and distributed on a de facto market, supported by permissive regulations concerning payment to donors (Almeling 2007; Spar 2007; Daniels and Heidt-Forsythe 2012). Similarly, substantial payment to participants in clinical research is permitted and routinely practised in several countries (Dickert and Grady 2008; Nuffield Council on Bioethics 2011). In the USA, fees can be high enough to enable healthy but poor individuals to make a living as "professional guinea pigs" (Abadie 2010), a phenomenon that reportedly also occurs in China and India (Cooper and Waldby 2014). Moreover, jurisdictions in, for example, India, Ukraine, Russia and some states in the USA permit commercial surrogacy arrangements, enabling a global fertility market (Waldby and Mitchell 2006; Svitnev 2010; Mohapatra 2012).[8] While all these practices have their critics and defenders, the selling framework has been most extensively and hotly debated with respect to an area where the gift model firmly holds sway: organ transplantation.[9]

Two main rationales are invoked to support the selling framework. The first appeals to efficiency. Many transplantable organs and tissues, kidneys in particular, are not available in sufficient quantities to satisfy all who would benefit from a transplant. As the matter is typically put, there is an "organ shortage": "demand" exceeds "supply". While different approaches to increasing supply have been tried with varying degrees of success, the most effective approach, it is argued, would be to offer donors (or their kin in cases of cadaveric donation) some form of economic incentive. Since people are more likely to donate for money than for free, a market system would make more organs available, saving and improving the lives of those who need them (Radcliffe-Richards *et al.* 1998; Wilkinson 2003; Matas 2004; Taylor 2005).

A market system is often thought to benefit not only recipients, but providers as well. The risks and burdens to donors or their kin vary greatly, depending on the organ in question, the quality of the care received, and so on. However, if the price is right, the argument goes, these risks and burdens may well be worth assuming for somebody in economic need. The organ sale is thus cast as a mutually beneficial exchange (Radcliffe-Richards *et al.* 1998; Taylor 2005).

The second main rationale for the selling framework appeals to the rights or autonomy of providers of body parts or bodily services. One version of the argument simply states that I own my body, and that I therefore have the right to use it as I see fit, which includes alienating parts of it in exchange for money (Andrews 1986). Other versions avoid the language of ownership, invoking providers' autonomy or liberty to the same effect: whether to accept money in exchange for their organs, tissues or bodily services is a choice that individuals themselves should be allowed to make (Fabre 2006; Wilkinson 2011). From this perspective, banning payment in order to protect providers is "paternalism in its worst form" (Savulescu 2003, 139).

A number of ethical concerns have been raised about the selling framework. One set of concerns targets the alleged efficiency of a market approach. For instance, in the transplantation context, some believe the introduction of monetary incentives would "crowd out" altruistically motivated donors, thus decreasing rather than increasing the supply of organs or tissues.[10] Others doubt that the benefits to living organ vendors would in fact outweigh the risks and burdens they face (Koplin 2014). Yet others argue that the health of recipients would be jeopardized because vendors would have an incentive to hide aspects of their lifestyle or medical history that would make their organs unsuitable for transplantation (Rothman and Rothman 2006; cf. Titmuss 1970).

Another set of concerns revolves around the autonomy or consent of providers of body parts or bodily services. A common worry about paying research participants is that a large sum of money may constitute an "undue inducement" capable of distorting their judgment, undermining the voluntariness of their consent or in other ways compromising their agency (Dickert and Grady 2008). Many research ethical guidelines therefore require payment to be kept at a modest level (FDA 1998; CIOMS 2002, §7). Similar concerns about the effect of money on people's decisions have been discussed in relation to paid organ donation (Wilkinson 2003) and paid gamete donation (Daniels and Heidt-Forsythe 2012). A distinct worry is that financial incentives may motivate third parties interested in providers' money to coerce or pressure the donor into the exchange (Satz 2010; Malmqvist 2014). Further, some argue that payment would disproportionally attract the very poor, who would not sell voluntarily because they would have no meaningful choice (Audi 1996).

Sometimes concerns about poverty are framed in terms of exploitation rather than, or in addition to, consent. Due to the limited options available to them, the argument goes, poor people are vulnerable to being taken advantage of in unfair or degrading ways when making their bodies available to others in return for payment (Widdows 2009; Panitch 2013).

Most importantly, perhaps, the selling framework runs up against deep and widespread beliefs about the non-commodifiability of the human body. The wrongness of reducing people's bodies, or certain of their body parts or bodily activities, to objects of market exchange is frequently asserted in the scholarly literature on bodily exchanges (Radin 1987; Cohen 1999; Sharp 2000) as well as in relevant policy documents. For instance, in its *Guiding Principles on Human Cell, Tissue and Organ Transplantation* the WHO states that payment for cells, tissues and organs "conveys the idea that some persons lack dignity and that they are mere objects to be used by others" (WHO 2010, 5). Often traced to Immanuel Kant's (1997 [1785]) famous dictum that persons should never be treated as means only but always also as ends in themselves, such assertions also invoke ideas about the market's instrumentalizing tendency and the essentiality of bodies to personhood.[11]

To accommodate different criticisms directed against the giving and selling frameworks, proponents of each have sought to refine their positions. For instance, in the organ donation context, advocates of the selling framework have proposed increasingly sophisticated forms of market regulation intended to prevent the alleged abuses of an unrestrained commerce (Erin and Harris 2003; Omar *et al.* 2010; Working Group on Incentives for Living Donation 2012). On the gift-giving side, recent decades have seen an increase in philosophical and theological interest in the meaning of giving, generosity and gratitude, and the (im)possibility and (un)desirability of gifts without returns

(Derrida 1997; Milbank 1999; Wyschogrod *et al.* 2002), and in critical sociological, anthropological and ethnological work on the gift metaphor in the transplantation context (Fox and Swazey 2002; Scheper-Hughes 2007; Shaw 2010). This has contributed to an expansion of the "conceptual toolkit for how to understand organ gifting" (Shaw 2015, 1; Zeiler 2014). Moreover, while rejecting outright payment, proponents of the gift framework have acknowledged the role of other incentives, such as public recognition and reimbursement of funeral expenses, as a way to increase donation rates (Delmonico *et al.* 2002). Notwithstanding these refinements of the giving and selling frameworks, the opposition between them continues to frame much contemporary scholarship on bodily exchanges in medicine.

Beyond giving and selling

There is a growing dissatisfaction with this oppositional framing of the debate. Based on an appreciation of the complexity of bodily exchanges in medicine, several scholars argue that the dichotomy between the giving and selling frameworks is misleading or false. Not only are healthcare and biomedical research increasingly areas where the same objects qualify as gifts at certain times and places and as commodities at others (Waldby and Mitchell 2006); but the oppositional framing also appears to imply that body parts and bodily services are provided and distributed only to help patients or only to secure a profit. Empirical research shows that providers' motivations are not that clear-cut (Pennings *et al.* 2014) and that the sale of bodily material can also be understood as helping others (Hoeyer 2009). Given these complexities, it is argued, accurately conceptualizing and evaluating bodily exchanges in medicine requires moving beyond seeing them as appropriately belonging to either category (Frow 1997; Callon 1998; Healy 2006; Almeling 2007; Waldby and Mitchell 2006; Hoeyer 2013).

In a recent report, the British Nuffield Council on Bioethics (2011) presents one of the more detailed efforts to move beyond the giving–selling dichotomy. Distinguishing itself from conceptualizations of bodily exchanges as properly belonging to either a commercial or a non-commercial sphere, the report describes an "Intervention Ladder" with six rungs ranging from simple information to potential providers to monetary incentives that leave providers financially better off. While interventions on the higher rungs involve money to an increasing degree, they may nonetheless be ethically acceptable in certain circumstances. On the face of it, this approach looks like a significant departure from the gift model. However, one may wonder whether it actually leaves the giving–selling distinction behind, or rather reaffirms it in different words. The report distinguishes "altruistic-focused interventions" intended to "stimulate people's altruistic motivations" (rungs one through four) from "non-altruistic-focused interventions" that encourage individuals who would not otherwise have considered donating to do so, sometimes by promising to improve their financial situation (rungs five and six). While the report states that the latter are not necessarily unethical, they are described as "ethically more complex" and as requiring special scrutiny. It would appear that the offer of money to providers remains at least *potentially* – though not, as in the gift model, *necessarily* – suspect. Otherwise, why the need for special scrutiny?

This volume shares the ambition to move beyond the giving–selling dichotomy. However, while not denying the insights of previous attempts to do so, it takes a different tack. In addition to probing the established giving and selling frameworks, the contributions to this volume provide material for sketching a distinct, far less familiar framework: that of *sharing*. In this framework, bodily exchanges are not conceptualized as momentary transactions between two parties wherein some good changes hands, but as temporally extended phenomena embedded in complex forms of relationality.

On the face of it, there are two reasons to believe that this alternative framing may prove illuminating. First, sharing is a broader category than both giving and selling in that it does not necessarily entail alienation and transfer. Unlike these other categories, it captures both practices that involve giving up and giving away part of one's body (organ and tissue donation) *and* practices that do not (surrogacy and research participation). This facilitates our inclusive take on bodily exchanges in medicine and allows insufficiently analysed similarities and differences between exchanges to emerge. Second, the notion of sharing escapes the opposition between the giving and selling frameworks. Unlike the former, it need not exclude the involvement of money in bodily exchanges; unlike the latter, it does not marginalize other-regarding motives among the parties to the exchange. It may therefore capture nuances commonly lost in the polarized debate between these frameworks, as well as accommodate practices that do not fit either of them.

In addition to these and other potential advantages of a sharing framework, however, there are also potential concerns. Rather than attempting to list the advantages and concerns here, we will let them emerge through the diverse analyses of bodily exchanges in medicine that the following chapters provide. In the concluding chapter, we draw on these contributions in order to sketch the sharing framework in greater detail and scrutinize its ethical implications.

Bodily giving, selling and sharing in this volume

In the first contribution to *Bodily Exchanges, Bioethics and Border Crossing*, Fredrik Svenaeus examines the ontological and ethical status of "exiled" body parts – i.e. organs, cells and tissues that have been removed from their site of origin in an individual human body. Drawing on phenomenological philosophy, Svenaeus argues that a biological perspective is insufficient for understanding what kind of things these body parts are. An adequate ontological analysis also needs to incorporate the perspectives of the persons from whom they are derived and the culture these persons live in. Svenaeus advances the term "sobject" to emphasize that bodily material divorced from one human body and not yet implanted into another neither qualifies as mere objects nor as part of a subject. Based on an examination of how different body parts relate to personal identity, he suggests that some sobjects matter more than others to the persons who exile or receive them. This analysis has important implications for ethical discussions about ownership over, and the giving or sharing of, bodily material. In this way, ethical analyses of bodily exchanges in medicine can benefit from proceeding in dialogue with ontological ones.

The next chapter, by Simone Bateman, also focuses on exiled body parts. More specifically, Bateman examines the case of surgically removed tissue that was once discarded as waste but that has proven increasingly capable of being transformed into valuable research specimens. Using Marcel Mauss' classic work on the gift as a heuristic tool, she shows how the scientific and commercial exploitation of these tissues challenges the gift-giving norm that is supposed to regulate the procurement and use of human body parts for research. The notion of the gift, she argues, implies robust requirements pertaining to informed consent and the protection of providers' privacy. However, these requirements have often been breached, as the well-known case of Henrietta Lacks demonstrates, and they are increasingly difficult to fulfil as tissue samples are used to gather growing quantities of genomic data that are useful in multiple forms of research and that may concern not only providers but also their relatives and descendants. Bateman ends by considering how present research practices would have to be modified in order to actually fit the ethical framework that allegedly governs them.

The following two chapters, by Erica Haimes and Leonardo de Castro, highlight another challenge to the gift framework: the involvement of money in bodily exchanges. Haimes' chapter explores the role of money from the perspective of donors involved in a UK "egg sharing" scheme, who receive reduced fees for their IVF treatment in return for providing eggs for somatic cell nuclear transfer research and research on avoiding the transmission of mitochondrial disease. This scheme is controversial because it has been perceived to be at odds with the restrictions imposed by European legislation on financial incentives to organ and tissue donors. Moreover, scholars have debated whether monetary offers "taint" or "crowd out" altruism or other values worth caring about. Haimes challenges the notion of money as one-dimensional, fungible entity that underlies these debates. Based on interviews with volunteers for the egg sharing scheme, she shows that money has variable contextual significances that tend to remain neglected in bioethical analyses. This inquiry enables a different set of distinctions to be drawn as regards the appropriateness and effects of money in relation to the body.

De Castro's chapter articulates a conception of sharing grounded in the Filipino concepts of *kagandahang loob* (good will), *utang na loob* (debt of good will) and *hiya* (moral shame) in order to provide a culturally informed account of organ donation. Through an elaboration on the difference between giving and sharing, de Castro questions the paradigm of non-remuneration in donation ethics, arguing that altruism need not always be defined in terms of the absence of payment or the expectation thereof. Furthermore, he argues that appreciating the ethical significance of particular acts of donation requires understanding the specific context where they are situated and the roles that individuals play in that context. Such understanding is needed for us to adequately grasp, and for transplant ethics committees to adequately respond to, the concerns of people who are hoping to have organ transplants approved. For de Castro, this approach enables a context-sensitive ethical discussion that gives some room for flexibility concerning the involvement of money without sacrificing general ethical principles.

In the next three chapters, Lesley A. Sharp, Sarah Jane Toledano and Kristin Zeiler continue the exploration of the notion of sharing in relation to bodily exchanges in medicine. Taking off from a discussion of sharing as a social act, Sharp examines what differentiates sharing from gift-giving, how scarcity might initiate sharing and how sharing can generate unusual, innovative and subversive acts. Her argument is developed through an analysis of two distinct yet related medical practices: human organ transfer and xenotransplantation – an experimental research area aimed at culling organs and tissues from different animal species for human use. Sharp uses the concept of sharing to highlight how human organ transfer can engender new forms of sociality as donor families and recipients reach out to each other and meet. In the xeno case, she shows how scientists, in response to seemingly insurmountable immunological hurdles and diminished funds, have established an "animal commons" of genetically modified pigs that are shared between labs. Sharp ends by asking what lessons these collective actions might inspire in the case of human organ transfer. More specifically, she considers whether altruistic donor chains – as a kind of "human commons" driven by a desire to share rather than by market logic – might be a viable response to the chronic scarcity of transplant organs.

Toledano examines the possibilities and limits of sharing the embodied experience of pregnancy in cases of surrogate motherhood. Engaging with Iris Marion Young's classic phenomenological work on pregnant embodiment, she seeks to move beyond the view of pregnancy as a dyadic maternal–foetal relationship. Whereas the pregnancy experience has often been conceptualized as being unsharable by those who are not, have not been or cannot become pregnant, Toledano questions whether this is so. Empirical studies of commercial and altruistic surrogacy suggest that others than the pregnant subject – in these cases the intended parents – are capable of sharing her experience in meaningful ways. However, this sharing is not only a potential source of mutual joy and support, but also harbours relational asymmetries and opportunities for transgression. Toledano's analysis demonstrates how assisted reproduction, though commonly criticized by feminists, can be a venue for rethinking taken-for-granted assumptions about pregnancy, embodiment and subjectivity.

Zeiler's chapter turns to the notion of giving-through-sharing that has previously been used to explore whether and how the donation of an organ (the giving) can be understood as an expression of the connectedness and continuity between the self and the other (the sharing) that is the very precondition of the self as embodied and situated in a world and in relations with others in phenomenological philosophy. She examines the potentially ethically problematic aspects of this basic form of sharing through a discussion of online organ solicitation and subsequent directed donation. Contrasting ethical concerns over online organ solicitation and donation with established ethical rationales for post-mortem and live donation to unknown recipients, and live donation between relatives and friends, Zeiler explores how this practice falls between common ways of thinking about donation ethics. She argues that online organ solicitation raises concern not only because it may allow donation queues to be sidestepped. It also brings to light how the social expression and sharing of meaning on pre-reflective levels of existence can enable us to be touched by and respond to the suffering of others in different ways, why the phenomenon of being touched needs to be acknowledged in ethics and why it evokes fundamental concerns.

While all the contributions to this volume engage with different forms of border crossing involved in bodily exchanges, the subsequent four chapters put special emphasis on the crossing of national borders. Donna McCormack's chapter examines how organ transplantation in fiction can raise ethical questions about migration, inequalities and postcolonial histories. Through an analysis of Malika Mokeddem's novel *The Forbidden Woman* – which narrates the medical doctor Sultana's return to the Algerian town she left behind long ago and the French kidney recipient Vincent's travel to his deceased donor's native Algeria in search of a post-transplant identity – McCormack explores the links between a colonial past and contemporary biotechnological practice. She argues that the novel makes manifest how transplantation and migration disrupt the linear temporalities demanded by national narratives and transplant professionals and renders apparent the self's emergence through the other. This provokes questions about how to live together despite hierarchical differences and how to remember silenced or unspoken histories.

Continuing on the transnational theme, Michael Humbracht, Insoo Hyun and Susanne Lundin engage with the phenomenon of stem cell travel, which occurs when patients travel to clinics abroad to receive unproven stem cell treatments. They argue that debates about how to combat this phenomenon have so far failed to appreciate the link between patient hope and autonomy and the importance of trust in medical authorities. A model of the doctor–patient relationship that moves beyond physician paternalism and patient consumerism is needed in order to manage the hope and spiritual distress that prompt patients to seek treatment abroad. The concept of sharing plays a dual role in the analysis that Humbracht and colleagues offer. Patients' willingness to share their cells with purveyors and their personal stories with each other online fuels this form of medical mobility. At the same time, the shared construction of treatment between doctors and patients, and in the future perhaps bodily sharing in the form of clinical trials, constitute ethically appropriate means of curbing it.

Focusing on the relocation of clinical trials to the developing world, Erik Malmqvist discusses whether benefiting from global injustice creates any special responsibility towards its victims. He argues that the poverty and lack of access to healthcare that often appear to motivate people in poor countries to enrol in research are deeply unjust. Because these conditions facilitate the development of drugs for patients in affluent countries, these patients appear to be the beneficiaries of injustice. This raises the question whether they have any special responsibility to improve these conditions – over and above the responsibilities they may have as citizens of rich democracies or consumers in a global economy. Malmqvist examines several justifications that philosophers have offered for attributing special responsibilities to the beneficiaries of injustice, finding all of them unhelpful in singling out these patients. The chapter ends by exploring the idea that the responsibility to address poverty and lack of access to healthcare in the developing world is in fact more widely shared.

The penultimate chapter, by Joseph Millum, also connects bodily exchanges in medicine to questions of global justice. Noting that many transnational exchanges (in medicine and elsewhere) occur between victims and beneficiaries of an unjust global order, Millum asks whether this background injustice should affect how these exchanges are evaluated. He considers three ways in which it might. First, power disparities between the parties may encourage the perception of wrongdoing even when no wrongdoing occurs. Second, the more powerful party is likely to have a duty to ameliorate injustice, which may be more effectively discharged by helping the less powerful party even though it is strictly speaking independent of their interaction. Third, background injustice makes the less powerful party vulnerable to exploitation. Expanding on this last issue, Millum discusses whether one can avoid exploiting somebody by providing benefits to other people – such as the communities from which participants in clinical trials are recruited. He argues that this idea makes sense in two cases: when the person is involved in a reciprocal relationship with these others and when she identifies with their interests.

The final chapter picks up and develops salient themes from the preceding chapters in order to outline a sharing framework for bodily exchanges in medicine. It is argued that this framework differs substantially from the more familiar giving and selling frameworks, in that it inspires a distinct type of ethical analysis. More precisely, it invites examination of the broader social and institutional context wherein bodily exchanges occur, and of their potential impact on parties beyond those immediately involved, bringing questions of distributive justice into focus. Moreover, the chapter argues that this framework avoids several common objections to the giving and selling frameworks, but also identifies abuses that it might be susceptible to. The chapter ends by pointing towards a few contested practical issues where a sharing framework might be a useful tool for ethical analysis.

Acknowledgements

The chapters in this volume were presented and discussed at the symposium *Sharing Bodies within and across Borders* at the Swedish Collegium for

Advanced Study, Uppsala University, in May 2014. We would like to thank the participants in the symposium for making it a successful event, the Collegium for hosting the symposium in its beautiful location, and *Riksbankens Jubileumsfond* (the Swedish Foundation for the Humanities and Social Sciences) and Linköping University for financial support. We are also grateful to participants in the Technology, Practice and Identity seminar at the Department of Thematic Studies: Technology and Social Change, Linköping University, for their input on drafts of the introductory and concluding chapters of this book.

Notes

1 Figure available at www.transplant-observatory.org/Pages/Facts.aspx.

2 Though routinely performed, blood transfusions are not unproblematic, as demonstrated by repeated scandals where recipients have been infected with, for example, hepatitis C or HIV (Feldman and Bayer 1999).

3 Bodily exchanges, as understood here, arguably occur in non-medical contexts as well, for instance in sexual activities. However, this volume focuses on the medical or healthcare setting. Not only do the bodily exchanges that occur in this setting seem unmatched in their variety and complexity. These exchanges are also facilitated and regulated by societal institutions in different ways, which makes ethical analysis and debate especially important.

4 In the first category we include practices where bodily material is appropriated in order to eventually be transferred back to providers themselves. This happens in autologous donation, where people "donate" cells or tissues to themselves to satisfy their own future health or reproductive interests (Waldby and Mitchell 2006), and in some forms of stem cell therapy. These practices raise similar issues as heterologous transfers since they also involve third parties that handle and may benefit from the provider's body parts in different ways.

5 Different versions of this view have been defended in regard to blood donation (Titmuss 1970), organ transplantation (Joralemon 1995; Delmonico *et al.* 2002), transplantation of cadaver tissue (Campbell 2004), clinical research (Chambers 2001) and the provision of tissue for biomedical research (Murray 1987). The works cited here constitute merely a small sample of the extensive medical, bioethical, philosophical and social scientific literature that endorses some variety of the gift framework.

6 www.skane.se/sv/Webbplatser/Skanes-universitetssjukhus/Organisation-A-O/Reproduktionsmedicinskt-centrum/Fertilitetsmottagningar/Spermadonation/Aggdonation.

7 This rationale is implicit in the assertion that organ donation is "generous" or "heroic" (see e.g. Participants in the International Summit on Transplant Tourism and Organ Trafficking 2008, 854, 856).

8 The description of these arrangements in terms of selling can been challenged as too simplistic. Empirical studies show that some women involved in paid forms of surrogate motherhood downplay business aspects and instead narrate surrogacy as a way to care for their own families (Pande 2009, 2010), frame their relationship to the commissioning parents in gift language (Teman 2010) and express hope that this relationship will last over time (Vora 2013).

9 Iran is often cited as an exception to the worldwide ban on organ sale, because its kidney transplantation system allows organ providers to receive a fixed amount from the state and a separate remuneration from the recipient or from a designated charitable organization (Hippen 2008). However, this arrangement has also been described as a case of rewarded gifting (Larijani *et al.* 2004).

10 Originally raised by Titmuss (1970) in relation to blood donation, this possibility has also been discussed in the organ donation setting (Rothman and Rothman 2006). There is some evidence from behavioural economics of crowding out effects in other contexts (Gneezy and Rustichini 2000).

11 Both of which have a long history in social and philosophical thought, the former stretching back at least to the founders of sociology (Zelizer 1997) and the latter to phenomenological thinkers such as Merleau-Ponty (2002 [1962]).

References

Abadie, R. 2010. *The Professional Guinea Pig: Big Pharma and the Risky World of Human Subjects.* Durham: Duke University Press.

Almeling, R. 2007. "Gender and the Medical Market in Genetic Material." *American Sociological Review* 72: 319–340.

Andrews, L. 1986. "My Body, My Property." *Hastings Center Report* 16(5): 28–38.

Audi, R. 1996. "The Morality and Utility of Organ Transplantation." *Utilitas* 8: 141–158.

Brännström, M., Johannesson, L., Bokström, H., Kvarnström, N., Mölne, J., Dahm-Kähler, P., Enskog, A., Milenkovic, M., Ekberg, J., Diaz-Garcia, C., Gäbel, M., Hanafy, A., Hagberg, H., Olausson, M., and L. Nilsson. 2015. "Livebirth after Uterus Transplantation." *The Lancet* 385: 607–616.

Callon, M. 1998. "Introduction: The Embeddedness of Economic Markets in Economics." In: *The Laws of the Markets*, edited by M. Callon, 1–57. Oxford: Blackwell.

Campbell, C.S. 2004. "The Gift and the Market: Cultural and Symbolic Perspectives." In: *Transplanting Human Tissue: Ethics, Policy, and Practice*, edited by S.J. Youngner, M.W. Anderson and R. Schapiro, 139–159. Oxford: Oxford University Press.

Chambers, T. 2001. "Participation as Commodity, Participation as Gift." *American Journal of Bioethics* 1(2): 48.

CIOMS (Council for International Organizations of Medical Sciences). 2002. *International Ethical Guidelines for Biomedical Research Involving Human Subjects.* Geneva: CIOMS/WHO.

Cohen, C.B. 1999. "Selling Bits and Pieces of Humans to Make Babies: *The Gift of the Magi* Revisited." *Journal of Medicine and Philosophy* 24: 288–306.

Cooper, M., and C. Waldby. 2014. *Clinical Labor: Tissue Donors and Research Subjects in the Global Bioeconomy.* Durham: Duke University Press.

Daniels, C.R., and E. Heidt-Forsythe. 2012. "Gendered Eugenics and the Problematic of Free Market Reproductive Technologies: Sperm and Egg Donation in the United States." *Signs* 37: 719–747.

Delmonico, F.L., Arnold, R., Scheper-Hughes, N., Siminoff, L.A., Kahn, J., and S.J. Youngner. 2002. "Ethical Incentives – Not Payment – for Organ Donation." *New England Journal of Medicine* 346: 2002–2005.

Derrida, J. 1997. *Given Time: 1. Counterfeit Money.* Chicago: University of Chicago Press.

Dickert, N., and C. Grady. 2008. "Incentives for Research Participants." In: *The Oxford Textbook of Clinical Research Ethics*, edited by E.J. Emanuel, C.C. Grady, R.A. Crouch, R.K. Lie, F.G. Miller and D.D. Wendler. New York: Oxford University Press.

Erin, C.A., and J. Harris. 2003. "An Ethical Market in Human Organs." *Journal of Medical Ethics* 29: 137–138.

Fabre, C. 2006. *Whose Body Is It Anyway? Justice and the Integrity of the Person.* Oxford: Oxford University Press.

FDA (Food and Drug Administration). 1998. Payment to Research Subjects – Information Sheet. Guidance for Institutional Review Boards and Clinical Investigators. Available at: www.fda.gov/RegulatoryInformation/Guidances/ucm126429.htm.

Feldman, E.A., and R. Bayer, eds. 1997. *Blood Feuds: AIDS, Blood, and the Politics of Medical Disaster.* Oxford: Oxford University Press.

Fox, R., and J. Swazey. 2002. *Spare Parts. Organ Replacement in American Society.* New York: Oxford University Press.

Frow, J. 1997. *Time and Commodity Culture: Essays in Cultural Theory and Postmodernity.* Oxford: Clarendon Press.

Gneezy, U., and A. Rustichini. 2000. "A Fine Is a Price." *Journal of Legal Studies* 29: 1–17.

Healy, K. 2006. *Last Best Gifts. Altruism and the Market for Human Blood and Organs.* Chicago: University of Chicago Press.

Hippen, B.E. 2008. "Organ Sales and Moral Travails: Lessons from the Living Kidney Vendor Program in Iran." *Policy Analysis* 28: 1–17.

Hoeyer, K. 2009. "Tradable Body Parts? How Bone and Recycled Prosthetic Devices Acquire a Price without Forming a 'Market'." *BioSocieties* 4: 239–256.

Hoeyer, K. 2013. *Exchanging Human Bodily Material: Rethinking Bodies and Markets.* Dordrecht: Springer.

Inhorn, M. 2011. "Globalization and Gametes: Reproductive 'Tourism,' Islamic Bioethics, and Middle Eastern Modernity." *Anthropology & Medicine* 18: 87–103.

Joralemon, D. 1995. "Organ Wars: The Battle for Body Parts." *Medical Anthropology Quarterly* 9: 334–356.

Kant, I. 1997 [1785]. *Groundwork of the Metaphysics of Morals.* Translated by M.J. Gregor. Cambridge: Cambridge University Press.

Koplin, J. 2014. "Assessing the Likely Harms to Kidney Vendors in Regulated Organ Markets." *American Journal of Bioethics* 14(10): 7–18.

Krolokke, C. 2014. "Eggs and Euros: A Feminist Perspective on Reproductive Travel from Denmark to Spain." *International Journal of Feminist Approaches to Bioethics* 7(2): 144–163.

Larijani, B., Zahedi, F., and E. Taheri. 2004. "Ethical and Legal Aspects of Organ Transplantation in Iran." *Transplantation Proceedings* 36: 1241–1244.

Lundin, S. 2015. *Organs for Sale. An Ethnographic Examination of the International Organ Trade.* Basingstoke: Palgrave Pivot.

Mahoney, J.D. 2000. "The Market for Human Tissue." *Virginia Law Review* 86: 163–223.

Malmqvist, E. 2014. "Are Bans on Kidney Sales Unjustifiably Paternalistic?" *Bioethics* 28: 110–118.

Matas, A.J. 2004. "The Case for Living Kidney Sales: Rationale, Objections and Concerns." *American Journal of Transplantation* 4: 2007–2017.

Mauss, M. 1967 [1923–1924]. *The Gift: Forms and Functions of Exchange in Archaic Societies.* Translated by I. Cunnison. New York: Norton.

Merleau-Ponty, M. 2002 [1962]. *Phenomenology of Perception.* Translated by Colin Smith. London: Routledge.

Milbank, J. 1999. "The Ethics of Self-Sacrifice." *First Things* 91: 33–38.

Mohapatra, S. 2012. "Achieving Reproductive Justice in the International Surrogacy Market." *Annals of Health Law* 21: 191–200.

Murray, T.H. 1987. "Gifts of the Body and the Needs of Strangers." *Hastings Center Report* 17(2): 30–38.

Nahman, M. 2012. *Extractions: Securing Borders/Trafficking Ova*. Basingstoke: Palgrave Macmillan.

Nuffield Council on Bioethics. 2011. *Human Bodies: Donation for Medicine and Research*. London: Nuffield Council on Bioethics.

Omar, F., Tufvesson, G., and S. Welin. 2010. "Compensated Living Kidney Donation: A Plea for Pragmatism." *Health Care Analysis* 18: 85–101.

Pande, A. 2009. "Not an 'Angel', not a 'Whore': Surrogates as 'Dirty' Workers in India." *Indian Journal of Gender Studies* 16: 141–173.

Pande, A. 2010. "Commercial Surrogacy in India: Manufacturing a Perfect 'Mother-Worker'." *Signs* 45: 969–992.

Panitch, V. 2013. "Surrogate Tourism and Reproductive Rights." *Hypatia* 28: 274–289.

Participants in the International Summit on Transplant Tourism and Organ Trafficking. 2008. "The Declaration of Istanbul on Organ Trafficking and Transplant Tourism." *Kidney International* 74: 854–859.

Pennings, G., de Mouzon, J., Shenfield, F., Ferraretti, A.P., Mardesic, T., Ruiz, A., and V. Goossens. 2014. "Socio-Demographic and Fertility-Related Characteristics and Motivations of Oocyte Donors in 11 European Countries including Supplementary File." *Human Reproduction* 29: 1076–1089.

Petryna, A. 2009. *When Experiments Travel: Clinical Trials and the Global Search for Human Subjects*. Princeton: Princeton University Press.

Radcliffe-Richards, J., Daar, A.S., Guttman, R.D., Hoffenberg, R., Kennedy, I., Lock, M., Sells, R.A., and N. Tilney. 1998. "The Case for Allowing Kidney Sales." *Lancet* 352: 1950–1952.

Radin, M. J. 1987. "Market Inalienability." *Harvard Law Review* 100: 1849–1937.

Rothman, S.M., and D.J. Rothman. 2006. "The Hidden Cost of Organ Sale." *American Journal of Transplantation* 6: 1524–1528.

Satz, D. 2010. *Why Some Things Should Not Be for Sale: The Moral Limits of Markets*. Oxford: Oxford University Press.

Savulescu, J. 2003. "Is the Sale of Body Parts Wrong?" *Journal of Medical Ethics* 29: 138–139.

Scheper-Hughes, N. 2003. "Rotten Trade: Millennial Capitalism, Human Values and Global Justice in Organ Trafficking." *Journal of Human Rights* 2: 197–226.

Scheper-Hughes, N. 2007. "The Tyranny of the Gift: Sacrificial Violence in Living Donor Transplants." *American Journal of Transplantation* 7: 507–511.

Schulz-Baldes, A., Biller-Andorno, N., and A.M. Capron. 2007. "International Perspectives on the Ethics and Regulation of Human Cell and Tissue Transplantation." *Bulletin of the World Health Organization* 85: 941–948.

Sharp, L. 2000. "The Commodification of the Body and Its Parts." *Annual Review of Anthropology* 29: 287–328.

Sharp, L.A. 2006. *Strange Harvest: Organ Transplants, Denatured Bodies, and the Transformed Self*. Berkeley: University of California Press.

Shaw, R. 2010. "Perceptions of the Gift Relationship in Organ and Tissue Donation: Views of Intensivists and Donor and Recipient Coordinators." *Social Science and Medicine* 70: 609–615.

Shaw, R. 2015. "Expanding the Conceptual Toolkit of Organ Gifting." *Sociology of Health and Illness*. Online early view DOI: 10.1111/1467-9566.12258.

Shimazono, Y. 2007. "The State of the International Organ Trade: A Provisional Picture Based on Integration of Available Information." *Bulletin of the World Health Organization* 85: 955–962.

Siminoff, L.A. and K. Chillag. 1999. "The Fallacy of the 'Gift of Life'." *Hastings Center Report* 29(6): 34–41.

Spar, D. 2007. "The Egg Trade – Making Sense of the Market for Human Oocytes." *New England Journal of Medicine* 356: 1289–1291.

Sque, M., Payne, S., and J. Macleod. 2007. "Gift of Life or Sacrifice? Key Discourses to Understand Organ Donor Families' Decision-making." *Mortality: Promoting the Interdisciplinary Study of Death and Dying* 11: 117–132.

Svenaeus, F. 2010. "The Body as Gift, Resource or Commodity? Heidegger and the Ethics of Organ Transplantation." *Journal of Bioethical Inquiry* 7: 163–172.

Svitnev, K. 2010. "Legal Regulation of Assisted Reproduction Treatment in Russia." *Reproductive Biomedicine Online* 20: 892–894.

Taylor, J.S. 2005. *Stakes and Kidneys: Why Markets in Human Body Parts Are Morally Imperative.* Aldershot: Ashgate.

Teman, E. 2010. *Birthing a Mother: The Surrogate Self and the Pregnant Self.* Berkeley: University of California Press.

Titmuss, R.M. 1970. *The Gift Relationship: From Human Blood to Social Policy.* London: Allen and Unwin.

Toledano, S.J., and K. Zeiler. 2016. "Hosting for the Others' Child? Relational Work and Embodied Responsibility in Altruistic Surrogate Motherhood." *Feminist Theory.*

Vora, K. 2013. "Potential, Risk, and Return in Transnational Indian Gestational Surrogacy." *Current Anthropology* 54: S97–S106.

Waldby, C., and R. Mitchell. 2006. *Tissue Economies. Blood, Organs, and Cell Lines in Late Capitalism.* Durham: Duke University Press.

Whittaker, A., and A. Speier. 2010. "'Cycling Overseas'. Care, Commodification, and Stratification in Cross-Border Reproductive Travel." *Medical Anthropology: Cross-Cultural Studies in Health and Illness* 29(4): 363–383.

WHO (World Health Organization). 2010. Guiding Principles on Human Cell, Tissue and Organ Transplantation. Available at: www.who.int/transplantation/Guiding_PrinciplesTransplantation_WHA63.22en.pdf.

Widdows, H. 2009. "Border Disputes across Bodies: Exploitation in Trafficking for Prostitution and Egg Sale for Stem Cell Research." *International Journal of Feminist Approaches to Bioethics* 2(1): 5–24.

Wilkinson, S. 2003. *Bodies for Sale: Ethics and Exploitation in the Human Body Trade.* London: Routledge.

Wilkinson, T.M. 2011. *Ethics and the Acquisition of Organs.* Oxford: Oxford University Press.

Working Group on Incentives for Living Donation. 2012. "Incentives for Organ Donation: Proposed Standards for an Internationally Acceptable System." *American Journal of Transplantation* 12: 306–312.

Wyschogrod, E., Goux, J.J., and E. Boynton, eds. 2002. *The Enigma of Gift and Sacrifice.* New York: Fordham University Press.

Zeiler, K. 2014. "Neither Property Right Nor Heroic Gift, Neither Sacrifice Nor Aporia – The Benefit of the Theoretical Lens of Sharing in Donation Ethics." *Medicine, Health Care and Philosophy* 17: 171–181.

Zelizer, V.A. 1997. *The Social Meaning of Money.* Princeton: Princeton University Press.

2 The lived body and personal identity

The ontology of exiled body parts

Fredrik Svenaeus

Introduction

In this chapter I will attempt to develop a phenomenology of parts of the human body that have been removed from their site of origin but nevertheless preserve their "aliveness". What happens when human body parts are stored in the medical laboratory and are even being transformed or cultivated there? How are we to view the ontological and ethical status of cells and organs that are being transplanted from one human body to another? Do these body parts preserve some kind of relationship to their source of origin: that is, the person from whom they have been retrieved? Do they *belong* to the person they originate from and, if so, in what way? What implications does this type of ownership have for ethical analysis? In some cases, at least, would the concept of *sharing* be more adequate to describe transfer of body parts between persons than the idea of a gift being made (Zeiler 2014)?

In order to understand what kind of object an exiled body part represents, it is not enough to study its biological makeup. An ontological analysis that incorporates the perspectives of the individual person and the culture she lives in is required. Matters regarding *identity* need to be taken into account in understanding what body parts represent for the people involved in exiling or receiving them. In this chapter I will turn to phenomenology in order to explore the ontology of the human body and with an emphasis on the thematic of exiled body parts. My aim is to move beyond biology and explore the implications that such an analysis may have for medical ethics.

Phenomenology of medicine and health care

Phenomenology is a tradition, more than one hundred years old, of studying and answering philosophical questions by proceeding from an analysis of lived experience; important classics are philosophers like Edmund Husserl, Martin Heidegger, Maurice Merleau-Ponty and Jean-Paul Sartre (Moran 2000). The starting point for the phenomenologist in understanding ontological issues is not the world of science but the meaning structures of the everyday world, that which the phenomenologist calls the "life world", or our "being-in-the-world". From the trunk that started growing in philosophy with Husserl and his successors at the beginning of the 20th century, contemporary phenomenology has branched out into many different disciplines. Scholars and researchers of art, literature, psychology, sociology, anthropology, pedagogy, history and, recently, also nursing and medicine, have tried to make use of phenomenology in investigating phenomena of concern in their field.

The main topic of the phenomenology of medicine and health care so far has been experiences and situations in which the *body* is insistently involved – experiences of phenomena such as illness, pain, disability, giving birth and dying (Toombs 2001; Slatman 2014; Zeiler and Folkmarson Käll 2014). In phenomenological analysis, ever since the days of Husserl, the body is most often assigned a place and function in every type of experience; however, the body may be more or less *invisible* to the person undergoing the experience in question. In most cases it remains in the background of our experience and our attention is, instead, focused on the things in the world that we are engaged with – reading a book, for instance. In some situations, however, the body "dys-appears" instead of disappearing, forcing us to take notice of its existence (Leder 1990). The experienced body can be a source of great joy, as when we enjoy a good meal, do sports, have sex or are just relaxing after a hard day of work. However, it can also be a source of great suffering to its bearer, when she falls ill and experiences pain, nausea, anxiety and other bodily ailments (Carel 2008; Svenaeus 2009).

The basic difference stressed in this context by the phenomenologist is between the body considered as a vehicle of human existence and the body considered as a biological organism, what is often referred to as a distinction between the "lived", versus the "living", body (Fuchs 2000; Gallagher 2005). When I have a headache, the pain in question invades my entire world – my attempts to concentrate, perceive, communicate, move and so on. If the doctors put me in a brain-scan machine, they may be able to detect processes going on in my brain and the rest of my body that are responsible for the pain, but they will never find my headache *experience*, the feel and meaning the pain has for me as a being-in-the-world, to speak in a phenomenological idiom. The living brain, representing the most important part of my living organism, does not equal the lived bodily perspective of the person, who feels, thinks and does things in the world together with others.

To suffer from a headache means to find oneself in a *first-person* perspective as regards the pain in question. To encounter another person having a headache means to perceive the headache from the *second-person* perspective: through the posture, gestures, facial expressions, ways of speaking and acting, etc., of the person in question. The *third-person* perspective on headache, on the other hand, in contrast to both the first- and the second-person perspective, is a perspective from a neutral party, who is interested in the biological, causal pathways that make the headache in question come into existence. We perceive other persons as directly connected to us through the lived expressions of their bodies, whereas our own body has an autonomous nature that is foreign to us in many ways and which can be studied by the doctor. Phenomenology starts out from the perspective of lived personal experience, but in this analysis it concerns the whole world of the embodied person, including the encounter with bodies of other persons and the possibility of taking a scientific perspective on any type of object appearing in view, including one's own body as a *living* thing, in this case studied by the very same *lived* body.

The difference between the first-person (and the second-person) and the third-person perspective on the body is an important one. It makes it possible to explain not only how human experience is meaningful and material simultaneously, but also how the body belongs to a person in a stronger and more primordial sense than a personal belonging such as a car or a house (Leder 1999; Svenaeus 2014). The body is not only ours, it is *us*. However, granted this phenomenological priority of bodily experience to all kinds of human activities, are all parts of the body equally important from the phenomenological point of view? The embodied brain clearly seems more important than the embodied leg from the vantage point of a person's being-in-the-world. Do we find other important differences on the phenomenological level when it comes to spelling out the meaning of different parts of the body, such as visceral organs, limbs, skin, various tissues, cells and DNA, for example? And how do these differences inform bioethical dilemmas within the field of organ and tissue transfer (Munson 2002; Campbell 2009; Svenaeus 2010)? These are questions I will address in this chapter.

Medical technology and exiled body parts

The new possibilities opened up by medical science and technology in controlling and transferring parts of the human body, in the last fifty years or so, have changed its ontology in many ways (for overviews, see Tilney 2003; Waldby and Mitchell 2006; Lock and Nguyen 2010). Parts of the human body attain new meaning and significance for us when medical science and technology make breakthroughs that are swiftly brought to our attention and often dramatized and hyped by the media in various ways (Liljefors *et al.* 2012). Medicine changes the perception and understanding of the human body in our contemporary culture. This is an ongoing process that can take new and sometimes unexpected turns. The scientific influence concerns new knowledge about the body and its parts – such as the working of DNA or the neural makeup of the brain, for instance – but above all, the influence is dependent upon what the scientific–technological inventions allow us to *do* with the body. If parts of the human body can be kept "alive" outside the human body in order to be transferred to another human body, or even be cultured by way of tissue engineering in the laboratory, how are we to understand the status of these parts? Do they belong to anybody? Do we owe some form of respect toward the bodily parts that we do not owe to other things in the world? What kind of things are they, really, and how do they relate to the individual human bodies from which they have originated in some way or another (Gunnarson and Svenaeus 2012)?

Klaus Hoeyer has recently suggested that we name such body parts, divorced from one human body and not yet implanted in another, "ubjects" (Hoeyer 2013, 5). Another suggestion, proceeding from a blending of "subject" and "object", would be "sobjects". Some kinds of tissues and organs have been in the "sobject zone" for a relatively long time: blood, bone and skin; more recently, other types of tissue and, also, the mother material of all types of possible tissues and organs, namely stem cells, have entered this domain (Waldby and Mitchell 2006; Liljefors *et al.* 2012; Cooper and Waldby 2014).

The medical manipulation of sobjects outside the human body makes it increasingly complicated to determine their origin and establish their ontological status. The procedure of somatic cell nuclear transfer, also referred to as therapeutic cloning, will, perhaps, make it possible to cultivate human cells of any type that are genetically identical to the patient receiving them. The technology, which is still at an experimental stage, proceeds by replacing the nucleus of an oocyte with the nucleus of a somatic cell in order to produce a stemcell line. This is done for therapeutic reasons, but the technology could also be used to produce a cloned embryo for reproductive purposes. The debates about cloning and stem cell research started after the announcement of the birth of Dolly the sheep in 1997 and they continue to be vibrant to the present day (Nussbaum and Sunstein 1999; Jensen 2014). However, the possibilities of transforming and creating various types of human cells have recently become even more stunning and complex. Somatic cells have been found to be reprogrammable; it is possible to turn them "backwards" and thus make them into stem cells – so-called "induced pluripotent stem cells" (Madonna 2012). The stem cells may then, if we become able to control their maturation, be developed into any type of human tissue. A piece of skin could become a brain, for example. Or, at least, to begin with, a skin cell could become a neuronal cell.

To grow brains in the laboratory may sound like nonsensical science fiction and it will probably never become a reality, considering the extremely complex organization of the billions of cells making up this organ. But stem cells that have been cloned, induced and/or genetically transformed by recombinant DNA or synthetic biology techniques could, in the future, also be used to produce gametes (Palacios-Gonzalez *et al.* 2014). By way of such techniques, somatic cells would be turned into oocytes or sperms that could give rise to new human beings. In these eventual cases we are talking not about cloning, but about a technological process by which every human being could become a mother or father (or both at the same time) transcending the present natural limits of human reproduction. My aim in this chapter is not to discuss all the ethical dilemmas that the above-mentioned cell-transforming technologies would give rise to if implemented in medical research and practice. My aim is simply to point out that the ontology of sobjects is changing quickly and is dependent on medical technologies that may take turns we are presently not even aware of.

If medical researchers become able to make neurons divide and develop into a human brain, in some way or another, the question of whose brain it is will in a sense become obsolete. It will, of course, be the brain of the person who feels, thinks and possibly acts by way of being embodied by it. And, by some other form of bodily extension, we should quickly add. The brain cannot stay in the vat; it needs more of a body to feel or think something in the first place, as brain scientists have been pointing out for a long time now (Damasio 2012). The neurosurgeon Robert J. White performed brain transplants on monkeys back in the 1970s, in which the experimental animals were able to see, hear and smell, but not move, for several days, according to the reports, and ever since these experiments took place, the possibility of transplanting a human head to a new body has been discussed (Canavero 2013). The important question in discussing brain transplants – that the monkeys were not able to answer – is how it feels to get a new body. Would one feel and think oneself to be the same person after the transplant or would the new bodily environment of the brain also change the identity of the person in question? How would the sex and history of the transplanted body affect the identity of the head that receives it? Will it become possible to connect brains to prosthetic bodies that are made out of non-biological tissue? Such questions are thrilling but impossible to answer at the present time.

In contrast to the contingent possibilities I have discussed above, sobjects presently found in the world most often have a clear point of origin and belonging. They come from an individual person, living or dead, and thus have a form of home that they have been *exiled* from. Sobjects are consequently body parts in exile that may find a new home – or be rejected and discarded – by being put into a new body, a body of another human being, who needs the body parts to heal and prosper in some way or another (Sharp 2006). These sobjects include blood, bone and skin cells, as well as a number of human organ and tissue types – kidney, heart, liver, lung, pancreas, uterus, hand and face – that can presently be transplanted (Gunnarson and Svenaeus 2012).

A special case, which I will return to below in more detail, is human germ cells, harvested and transferred, and embryos created in vitro. However, granted that sperms and eggs and embryos are best described as "exiled" when they leave one human body to be implanted in another, they are, indeed, exiled in ways that are peculiar to the history, logic and new technological possibilities of a very old human practice: procreation. Sex and childbirth have a far longer history than blood transfusion and organ transplantation, and this must be kept in mind when doing an ontology of gamete sobjects.

In doing an ontology of sobjects, and in exploring the ways such an analysis has implications for ethics, I think we must take into consideration distinctions between different *kinds* of body parts that can be exiled, manipulated and cultivated by researchers and doctors in the ways I have described above.

However, this analysis cannot remain medical in the sense that biological facts about how body parts work, and how we can control them by technological means, would be the only relevant information to consider. The body, as the phenomenologist points out, is a lived, meaningful dimension that extends into human society and culture. How can the phenomenology of the lived body inform the ontology of sobjects? To this question I now turn.

The ontology of the lived body and its parts

Returning to the issue of embodiment viewed from the phenomenological first-person perspective, it is crucial to point out that the lived body does not appear as a sum of perceived parts, but rather consists in an experience of wholeness and transparency. The lived body is not the lived kidney plus the lived heart plus the lived face plus the lived hands plus the lived legs, and so on. The lived body is a kind of perceptual scheme: a pattern and structure of meaning that makes it possible to feel, perceive, and even imagine and think about, what things are like in the world (Leder 1990; Gallagher 2005). And, still, it is undoubtedly the case that different body parts carry different meaning and significance from the first-person perspective (Svenaeus 2012; Slatman 2014). The kidney does not partake in the lived body in the same way as the hand does. The body parts in question have not only different biological functions, but also different phenomenological significance. This significance is a result not only of the experiences we have of our own body in a direct way – when the stomach hurts or the legs feel jumpy, for instance – but also of the ways we are perceived and understood by others. The first-person perspective includes the second-person perspective, since we are always situated in a shared life world (Zahavi 2005). The phenomenological significance of my face cannot be divorced from the being-in-the-world I share with other persons, who perceive and interpret my appearance and identity in various ways (Perpich 2010). When I look at myself in the mirror, I do so in a world in which the presence of other persons is already taken for granted and makes the idea of an outer appearance possible in the first place.

We can, I believe, spell out the phenomenological differences between kinds of body parts by stressing either what parts are most essential from the point of view of the *health and survival* of the person or from the point of view of the *personal identity* of the person. The health and survival point of view overlaps more or less with a biological understanding of the body, whereas the identity issue is determined by the affective and perceptual schemas of the lived body that are extended into the meaning-shaping patterns of society and culture (Fuchs 2013). Not only our outer appearance but also the outlook on our internal parts are culturally impregnated, the most obvious example of this being the heart. The heart is traditionally considered as the origin of the feelings, identity and moral stature of a person, not only as a pump of blood necessary for our survival. In some situations we may also consider parts of our bodies as *foreign* elements that are *not* proper parts of us and that we want to get rid of. Most people do not identify strongly with their potbellies, and they may look forward to having them removed through plastic surgery. A kidney or leg that no longer serves its function and makes the person ill or disabled may be viewed as a defective and strange thing that prevents the person from being at home with her own body (Svenaeus 2012). Some people even want to amputate healthy limbs to feel more at home with themselves, a psychiatric disorder known as Body Integrity Identity Disorder (BIID) (Sullivan 2014). We identify more and less strongly with our bodily looks and the way our bodies perform, and the reasons for this may be cultural as well as biological.

What kind of *general patterns* do we find regarding the meaning and importance of various body parts for our personal identity (in a positive as well as a negative sense)? One would assume that the *size* of the body part should be important. It does not matter so much to me as a person if I lose a couple of hair or skin cells: as a matter of fact, I do this all the time, even right now writing this chapter, whereas the sudden chopping off of my legs would mean a great deal to me, as regards not only my wellbeing but also my personal identity. My legs mean much more to me than a piece of skin or some hairs from my head. My legs probably mean more to me than all the hairs on my head, but if we start talking about large areas of my skin, the competition becomes more evenly matched. Massive skin-tissue damage from burning would be not only exceedingly painful, but also personality transforming in the sense of changing my looks and abilities to do things in the world, just as is the case with the double leg amputation. It is not only the number of cells that count, however, but where they are located and how they perform their bodily functions related to the capacities of the lived body. Ten thousand brain cells in a certain location may be significant in a way that another ten thousand cells are not, whether in the brain, lungs or kidneys. And types of tissue that regenerate more easily and more spontaneously, and that we often lose as part of a natural process – blood, skin, hair, nails – are generally less important to us than tissues that do not regenerate easily – neurons or heart muscle tissue, for example.

Separating the *inner* and *outer* dimensions of our lived bodies is another possibility for distinguishing the meaning and significance of body parts from the phenomenological point of view. I can see and move my hands, arms, feet, legs, belly, butt, sexual organs, ears, eyes, nose, mouth and everything else that is visible to me. Underneath my skin, on the other hand, we find a fleshy and bloody, rather unknown, realm that we are unfamiliar with except for sensory perceptions that make it possible for me (at least at some points) to *feel* my heart, lungs, intestines and so on. We do not recognize our inner organs from their *looks* as being ours. As a matter of fact, we rarely take a look at the insides of human beings (or other animals) at all, if we are not doctors, butchers, or belong to some other peculiar profession. Inner organs are foreign and uncanny to us in ways that outer organs and limbs are not (Nancy 2008; Shildrick 2014). And despite this, our visceral life is immensely important to us from the lived perspective, especially at the point of becoming problematic in causing us pain or other bodily discomfort. We feel the inner organs when they fail us, and this is an alienating experience since it hits us at the very core of our existence (Leder 1990; Svenaeus 2009, 2014; Slatman 2014). Yet this importance is anonymous in nature in the sense that the body parts are not individually recognized by way of perception, but rather are responsible for a general discomfort or, in other cases, positive feeling of wellbeing (Zeiler 2010).

Proceeding from the division of the inner and the outer, I would say that my hand is much more personal to me than my kidney is. The thought of having one's hands, feet, penis or face removed after one's death to be incorporated in the lived body of another person would probably cause most people far more concern and second thoughts than having one's kidneys, lungs, liver or heart transplanted. Likewise, the use of one's DNA to clone another human being would be problematic to most people in a way that using blood or bone marrow from one's living or dead body to help other persons in need would not. The way a person perceives and understands different body parts as related to her personal identity and the way she feels about their being transplanted and received by others may vary a lot, however, depending on the basic cultural values a person embodies and believes in. Religious beliefs can play a large role here, and so can the belief in medical science and technological progress as a kind of metaphysical and moral outlook.

Given the fact that the perceived personal identity of body parts may vary on a scale from having absolutely no significance apart from sustaining the health and life of a person, to every body part being associated with personal identity in a strong sense – depending on the culturally instituted meaning patterns informing a person's understanding of the essence of personhood – I have discussed in this section ways that different body parts are typically found to be more or less important for our personal identity (see also Svenaeus 2012). In this discussion, the size distinction has been found to be insufficient, whereas the inner–outer distinction has proved to be more promising. In order to carry on the phenomenological analysis of the meaning of lived and exiled body parts, I will now deepen a thematic that has already been addressed above, namely, the way medical knowledge and technology impregnate the cultural meaning of our bodies in the contemporary life world. Popularized medical science has to a large extent replaced religious understandings of the human body and its parts in the secularized world of the twenty-first century.

Medical science, phenomenology and culture

Medical science and technology are, as discussed above, certainly very important to body ontology. Biological processes make our lives possible and determine the limits of what we can experience and do in the world, and even what we can think and imagine to be there. New medical–technological inventions that can assist us when the body fails, or even extend our natural possibilities, are, as a consequence of this, essential for body-part ontology (Gordijn and Chadwick 2008). But as I have also pointed out, biological processes and medical knowledge are not the *only* things that matter to a human life, and *how* they matter will depend on how they are lived and interpreted in human culture. The lived dimension starts out from bodily experiences, but as soon as the person begins to act and reflect in a world shared with other persons, cultural processes will be significant in determining the meaning of medical knowledge and technologies. The lived body is culturally *extended* and, also, culturally *impregnated* by human beliefs and our search for meaning and understanding in a shared life world.

This is perhaps most obvious when we enter the domain of human body parts that have been "exiled" and are kept in between bodies. The symbolic significance of a heart or a brain or a hand is never more visible than when placed on a table or tray of polished metal, displayed in a kind of iconic way to our horrified and yet mesmerized gazes. Parts of organs that we do not recognize immediately, or cultures of cells that are barely visible to us in petri dishes, can be made equally iconic, but in order for this to happen they need to be put under the microscope and made more visible and understandable by way of medical–technological tools that guide our gazes in various ways. Think about a sperm and oocyte uniting to form an embryo in the petri dish, or about the strains of nucleotides forming the molecule of DNA, as they are being portrayed in pictures accompanying various attempts to tell stories of medical success.

In the analysis above, we saw how the lived perspective on the body allowed us to discern a certain priority connected to the *visibility* of parts of the body that may be put into exile. Prioritizing by size, in contrast to the inner–outer distinction, did not work well as a guide in determining priority of body parts; the thing that ultimately matters is rather what type of organ or tissue we are discussing and how it performs its function in the whole organism. The size distinction is also problematic in that it does not acknowledge that what is nowadays exceedingly important for our personal identity is what we find in the *nucleus* of every single cell of ours. I am talking about DNA, of course, the parts of our bodies that make, not only in a biological sense, but nowadays also in a cultural sense, the fleshy material that I consist of *mine* (Frank 2011).

Medical science and technology have a deep impact on cultural understanding in the contemporary world, and these scientific–cultural patterns inform the experiences and understandings of our bodies. When people feel and claim that cells that have been cultivated in the laboratory *belong* to them, it is because the cells in question contain their unique DNA. I am increasingly my DNA. Actually, I suspect that it is only the brain – remember my previous example – that beats the DNA in the cultural identity race of our day. To remove parts of the heart, liver or lungs of a person will be much more important from the point of view of wellbeing and survival than the changing of some rather inessential part of the strings of DNA in our cells. Yet from the point of view of identity, I think many persons would perceive such a change by way of gene therapy as far more identity changing. The heart is increasingly just a pump, whereas the DNA is increasingly me. The lived perspective of phenomenology must include this scientific–cultural impact on the meaning patterns of the life world, also and especially when this impact concerns the nature of our embodiment and our personal identity.

In discussing the importance of our personal genome from the point of view of identity, we also need to consider the ontological status of gametes – oocytes and sperms. Sperms, in the old-fashioned, traditional form of procreation, were exiled only to more or less immediately fuse with an egg cell in the body of a woman or to be wasted there – leaving aside the case of masturbation and sexual activities that do not result in ejaculation in the vagina. Oocytes have only more recently become sobjects in the practice of in vitro fertilization (IVF). The possibilities of storing and using gametes in IVF and associated research practices have clearly changed their ontology and importance to us in many ways. Gametes have become carriers of our personal identity, which can eventually become realized in giving rise to babies created by way of medical–technological assistance. Biological parenthood, in one way, is becoming increasingly insignificant, since men and women may have hundreds of children they have never met but have given rise to through donating or selling gametes. On the other hand, IVF has not only made having children possible for couples or individuals who are unable to become parents in the traditional way; it has also reinforced the importance of having children that are genetically related to the parents. Couples and individuals use IVF not only to have children rather than not having any; they use IVF to make sure their children are genetically their *own*, rather than genetically foreign to them, as in the case of adoption (Cooper and Waldby 2014).

Five criteria in doing sobject ontology

In accordance with the phenomenological analysis developed above, I think a person will have stronger claims to control, and also reasons to be concerned about, what may happen to parts of her body that are (1) necessary for her continued health and survival, (2) not spontaneously regenerated in the body when removed, (3) culturally and/or scientifically taken to be essential for personal identity, (4) expressive of her perceived personality in a world shared with others and (5) made use of in ways that express the specific genetic setup of the sobject.

Criterion one targets the organs we cannot remove without ruining the health or terminating the life of a person. This first criterion does not apply in the case of brain-dead persons because these persons are no longer alive and cannot be healthy or ill. A person may be concerned about what happens to her body parts after she is dead, but in this case criteria three, four or five are applicable, not number one. Criterion two is supposed to reflect the fact that we are less concerned about losing types of cells that regenerate spontaneously when removed from our body, such as blood and hair cells. We may still be concerned about regenerative types of cells being used in reproduction (sperm) or placed in or on the bodies of other persons (blood, hair), but in these cases, criteria four and five are the ones to explore. Criterion three targets the priority of the brain and, historically, organs such as the heart and the blood as central for personhood and identity. In contemporary Western secularized societies the heart or blood do not in most cases qualify as essential for personhood, but they have done so historically, and they may do so in other cultural settings. Criterion four concerns faces, hands (arms), feet (legs) and, also, genitals – parts of the body that are visible to us and other persons. Criterion five, finally, is supposed to handle the importance we invest in our specific genetic setup, not least in the case of gametes.

The fifth criterion is formulated by adding the assumption that the sobject in question is *used* in a particular way after being removed from the body. We do not care much about sperms lost in masturbation or about oocytes that are not fertilized, or even about embryos that do not get implanted in the womb (I will not go into details of different types of contraceptive measures and early forms of abortion here). In a sense, this use-assumption is taken for granted in the case of the other criteria as well, since the body part, in being removed, is assumed to be made into a sobject; that is, it is being kept "alive" either in the laboratory or in another human body. The first criterion is not formulated out of a concern for identity-transgressing issues and thus, in a sense, it may be superfluous in the present analysis. That we care the most about cells and organs that we cannot lose without also losing our health or life is simply a matter of the body parts *being removed from* our body, not about their being transplanted into another body. We would be equally concerned, and in an equal way, if the body parts stayed in our body but ceased to perform their proper biological functions. The remaining four criteria also address the issue of what happens when the body part that is removed takes on a new "life" in the laboratory or in the body of another human being.

As I have also touched upon, medical technology may make the distinctions between different types of body parts obsolete by manipulating sobjects in ways that make them change and grow into things they were originally not. Nevertheless, I think our contemporary intuitions about the ways in which sobjects are essential for our health and survival and our personal identity are taken into account by the five criteria listed above. The fulfilling of one or more of these five criteria will mean that the sobject in question is *attached* to a person's lived body and identity in a way that other sobjects are not to an equal degree. In the same way, a person who receives sobjects that fulfil one or more of the criteria has stronger reasons to care about their origin than in the case of other sobjects. And the reason to care becomes greater if two criteria are fulfilled rather than one. A kidney does not regenerate if it is removed, but on the other hand it is not necessary for continuing a healthy life if proper aftercare is provided (criterion one) and it is not perceived as central for personal identity and personhood (criterion three). Body parts such as the heart and hand fulfil two criteria (numbers one and two, and numbers two and four, respectively), whereas the brain appears to be the only organ fulfilling three criteria in contemporary Western society (one, two and three).

Strong-identity-bearing sobjects and ethics

In what ways does distinguishing "strong-identity-bearing sobjects", if I may call them so, have repercussions for the way we think about the relationships established between persons by the transfer of body parts (Svenaeus 2012)? I think the reasons for resisting a view of sobjects as only biological resources and commodities on a market are even stronger in these cases than in others (Svenaeus 2010). Strong-identity-bearing sobjects (SIBS) are different from other sobjects in that they are closer to the core and essence of an individual person than other sobjects are. However, this ontological distinction made from the phenomenological perspective could be interpreted in various ways when it comes to the ethics of organ and tissue transfer (see also Svenaeus 2014).

In formulating the criteria of SIBS above, I used the expression "a person will have stronger claims to control, and also reasons to be concerned about, what may happen to parts of her body that …". This implies that the individual claims of the person giving up body parts turned into sobjects are stronger when one or several of the criteria are applicable. If, for instance, cells, tissues or organs harvested in the process of research are used to do things other than what the person consented to when donating, and this use involves turning them into SIBS, the reasons to oppose such use will be even stronger than in the case of weak-identity-bearing sobjects (WIBS). The main criterion involved in this case is presently number five. If I donate sperm for research and this sperm is instead used in IVF, my claims to control what happens to the cells in question appear to have been disregarded to a much larger degree than if I donate sperm for research and the sperm is used in research procedures that I have not consented to but that do not involve turning the cells into SIBS.

Commodification is particularly problematic when we are dealing with SIBS, and so is resourcification in the sense that the body parts could be viewed as parts of an anonymous, biological machinery only. But the fact that SIBS, such as brains, hearts, faces, kidneys and gametes, are more firmly tied to personal identity than blood cells and skin cells are, is not necessarily an argument for or against making WIBS public resources or commodities on a market. Everything that originates in the living and lived body has some sort of personal connection to it through its place of origin, so the need to involve the origin-person in harvesting sobjects will not be insignificant in these cases, either. Nevertheless, WIBS are more similar to ordinary "non-alive" commodities than SIBS are. The analysis and distinguishing of SIBS in contrast to WIBS may indeed be important, since the argument that some things should not be sold *simply* because they consist of human cells will probably be found increasingly less convincing in the biotech future, especially when we become even more able to manipulate or even artificially produce such cells in the laboratory (Campbell 2009). The treatment of SIBS demands different ethical considerations than the treatment of human, biological material as such.

To donate SIBS will create bonds between giver and receiver to a larger degree than in the case of WIBS, since identity issues are involved in a more thorough sense (Campbell 2009; Sharp 2006). To acknowledge these more- or less-strong-identity issues in the philosophical and bioethical analysis and debate, we would do better to describe and name the situations of organ, tissue and cell harvesting in the case of SIBS as a form of *sharing*, than as a form of giving. A person shares parts of herself rather than gives away parts of herself in the cases of SIBS donation, because the parts that are transferred from one body to another are tied to the *identity* of the donor. This does not mean that the receiver of a transplant in standard cases inherits parts of the donor's personality in the transfer of SIBS, as in living kidney donation or in deceased donation of organs such as the heart, lung or liver. The exception to this (in the future) would be brain transplants and also, possibly, present or future cases of transplanting "outer" parts, such as the face and hand. Another exception in which personality transfer is a real issue are cases of SIBS procedures involving the expression of DNA in procreative measures giving rise to offspring.

However, the strong-identity issues involved in transplanting inner organs are better understood as giving rise to, or strengthening, bonds *between* persons than as transferring personality traits. When we share ourselves with others in transplanting SIBS we become connected in a way that resembles the way families are formed by way of procreation (Svenaeus 2010). The bonds in question are not entirely of the same type, certainly, but they represent forms of bodily *sharing* that tie people together in altruistic and *caring* ways. It is possible, certainly, to have children only in the interest of strengthening and widening one's own influence in the world, just as it is possible to "donate" organs in exchange for money (the organ and tissue trade), but in most (and laudable) cases the care felt and shown for the child or patient in need will contribute to non-selfish bonds being formed when sharing SIBS. The idea of *sharing* exiled body parts in this way appears to be a promising alternative to the standard metaphors of giving or trading in medical ethics (Zeiler 2014).

Conclusion

The phenomenological idea that we belong to our own bodies in a fundamental way, rather than the other way around, can work as an antidote to the influential organ-commodity paradigm in contemporary bioethics. The phenomenological account can deliver an argument explaining why body parts are not just another type of thing to be traded, but rather are fundamental parts of our self-being. We are born *as* a body coming from *another* body. The body makes our existence and appearance as persons possible, and it does so in a way that is related to how we depend on each other as finite human beings living in the world. This explains why organs are not things that belong to us in the same way as things in the outer world do. Organs are identity bearing in the sense that they belong to the *processes* of selfhood – the lived body – rather than being things that the person controls and makes decisions about. Therefore, according to an embodied, phenomenological view, organs should not be traded, even though they can and should be shared by way of transplants. "Giving life", as the slogan for encouraging organ donation goes, is a *sharing* of life, not an offer of a valuable commodity. Rather than fearing that a view of parts of the body as anything more than useful biological material will create confusion and feelings of guilt in patients who receive new organs, health care professionals should acknowledge to a greater extent the bonds that are being created between people and families by organ transplantation, and also in cases of posthumous transplantation. The same goes for donation of gametes in which an instrumentalized and commodified view of the practice of having babies could be countered by the phenomenological argument of strong-identity bonds.

References

Campbell, A. V. 2009. *The Body in Bioethics.* London: Routledge.

Canavero, S. 2013. "HEAVEN: The Head Anastomosis Venture Project Outline for the First Human Head Transplantation with Spinal Linkage (GEMINI)." *Surgical Neurology International* 4, Suppl S1: 335–342.

Carel, H. 2008. *Illness: The Cry of the Flesh.* Stocksfield: Acumen Publishing.

Cooper, M., and C. Waldby. 2014. *Clinical Labor: Tissue Donors and Research Subjects in the Global Bioeconomy.* Durham and London: Duke University Press.

Damasio, A. 2012. *Self Comes to Mind: Constructing the Conscious Brain.* London: Vintage Books.

Frank, L. 2011. *My Beautiful Genome: Exposing Our Genetic Future.* Oxford: Oneworld Publications.

Fuchs, T. 2000. *Leib, Raum, Person: Entwurf einer phänomenologischen Anthropologie.* Stuttgart: Klett-Cotta.

Fuchs, T. 2013. "The Phenomenology of Affectivity." In: *The Oxford Handbook of Philosophy and Psychiatry*, edited by K.W.M. Fulford, M. Davies, R.G.T. Gipps, G. Graham, J.Z. Sadler, G. Stanghellini and T. Thornton, 612–631. Oxford: Oxford University Press.

Gallagher, S. 2005. *How the Body Shapes the Mind.* Oxford: Oxford University Press.

Gordijn, B., and R. Chadwick, eds. 2008. *Medical Enhancement and Posthumanity.* Dordrecht: Springer.

Gunnarson, M., and F. Svenaeus, eds. 2012. *The Body as Gift, Resource, and Commodity: Exchanging Organs, Tissues, and Cells in the 21st Century.* Huddinge: Södertörn Studies in Practical Knowledge.

Hoeyer, K. 2013. *Exchanging Human Bodily Material: Rethinking Bodies and Markets.* Dordrecht: Springer.

Jensen, E.A. 2014. *The Therapeutic Cloning Debate: Global Science and Journalism in the Public Sphere.* Farnham Surrey: Ashgate Publishing.

Leder, D. 1990. *The Absent Body.* Chicago: University of Chicago Press.

Leder, D. 1999. "Whose Body? What Body? The Metaphysics of Organ Transplantation." In: *Persons and Their Bodies: Rights, Responsibilities, Relationships*, edited by M.J. Cherry, 233–264. Dordrecht: Kluwer.

Liljefors, M., Lundin, S., and A. Wiszmeg, eds. 2012. *The Atomized Body: The Cultural Life of Stem Cells, Genes and Neurons.* Lund: Nordic Academic Press.

Lock, M., and V.-K. Nguyen. 2010. *An Anthropology of Biomedicine.* Malden, MA: Wiley-Blackwell.

Madonna, R. 2012. "Human-Induced Pluripotent Stem Cells: In Quest of Clinical Applications." *Molecular Biotechnology* 52(2):193–203.

Moran, D. 2000. *Introduction to Phenomenology.* London: Routledge.

Munson, R. 2002. *Raising the Dead: Organ Transplants, Ethics and Society.* Oxford: Oxford University Press.

Nancy, J.-L. 2008. "The Intruder." In: *Corpus*, edited by J.-L. Nancy, 161–173. New York: Fordham University Press (original work published 2000).

Nussbaum, M.C., and C.R. Sunstein, eds. 1999. *Clones and Clones: Facts and Fantasies about Human Cloning.* New York: Norton.

Palacios-Gonzalez, C., Harris, J., and G. Testa. 2014. "Multiplex Parenting: IVG and the Generations to Come." *Journal of Medical Ethics* 40: 752–758.

Perpich, D. 2010. "Vulnerability and the Ethics of Facial Tissue Transplantation." *Journal of Bioethical Inquiry* 7: 173–185.

Sharp, L.A. 2006. *Strange Harvest: Organ Transplants, Denatured Bodies, and the Transformed Self.* Berkeley: University of California Press.

Shildrick, M. 2014. "Visceral Phenomenology: Organ Transplantation and Identity." In: *Feminist Phenomenology and Medicine*, edited by K. Zeiler and L. Folkmarson Käll, 47–68. New York: SUNY Press.

Slatman, J. 2014. *Our Strange Body: Philosophical Reflections on Identity and Medical Interventions.* Amsterdam: Amsterdam University Press.

Sullivan, N. 2014. "'BIID'? Queer (Dis)orientations and the Phenomenology of 'Home'." In: *Feminist Phenomenology and Medicine*, edited by K. Zeiler and L. Folkmarson Käll, 119–142. New York: SUNY Press.

Svenaeus, F. 2009. "The Phenomenology of Falling Ill: An Explication, Critique and Improvement of Sartre's Theory of Embodiment and Alienation." *Human Studies* 32: 53–66.

Svenaeus, F. 2010. "The Body as Gift, Resource, or Commodity? Heidegger and the Ethics of Organ Transplantation." *Journal of Bioethical Inquiry* 7: 163–172.

Svenaeus, F. 2012. "Organ Transplantation and Personal Identity: How Does Loss and Change of Organs Affect the Self?" *Journal of Medicine and Philosophy* 37: 139–158.

Svenaeus, F. 2014. "Organ Transplantation Ethics from the Perspective of Embodied Selfhood." In: *The Routledge Companion to Bioethics*, edited by J. Arras, E. Fenton and R. Kukla, 570–580. London: Routledge.

Tilney, N.L. 2003. *Transplant: From Myth to Reality.* New Haven: Yale University Press.

Toombs, S. K., ed. 2001. *Handbook of Phenomenology and Medicine.* Dordrecht: Kluwer.

Waldby, C., and R. Mitchell. 2006. *Tissue Economies: Blood, Organs, and Cell Lines in Late Capitalism.* Durham and London: Duke University Press.

Zahavi, D. 2005. *Subjectivity and Selfhood: Investigating the First-Person Perspective.* Cambridge, MA: MIT Press.

Zeiler, K. 2010. "A Phenomenological Analysis of Bodily Self-Awareness in the Experience of Pain and Pleasure: On Dys-Appearance and Eu-Appearance." *Medicine, Health Care and Philosophy* 13(3): 333–342.

Zeiler, K. 2014. "Neither Property Right nor Heroic Gift, Neither Sacrifice nor Aporia: The Benefit of the Theoretical Lens of Sharing in Donation Ethics." *Medicine, Health Care and Philosophy* 17(2): 171–181.

Zeiler, K., and L. Folkmarson Käll, eds. 2014. *Feminist Phenomenology and Medicine.* New York: SUNY Press.

3 Putting the gift relationship to test

The peculiar case of research on discarded human tissue

Simone Bateman

Introduction

Human biological materials (such as blood, saliva, urine, faeces, etc.), and in particular what has long been known as discarded tissue (biopsies, surgically removed tumours, aborted embryos and foetuses, placentas, etc.), have been used for research purposes over many decades. Their use may initially appear unproblematic: most of these tissues, with the exception of embryos and foetuses, are not considered intrinsically valuable and many are constantly renewed by the body. Others are potentially lethal so that surgically removing them is not controversial; and until recently, when these tissues are separated from the body, they are not easily identifiable with the donor. These very characteristics, as well as the fact that most of these tissues can be collected without harming the provider, have led regulators in many countries to exempt research on human tissue from institutional oversight.

And yet, the scientific practices associated with the full exploitation of these human materials, and in particular cell-culturing and cryopreservation, have transformed what was once discarded tissue (also known today as "residual tissue") into potentially valuable research specimens that can be easily stored for long periods of time and shipped to research teams all over the world – sometimes well beyond the death of the donor – for use in multiple research projects. These projects generate not only knowledge but also profits for research teams and their industrial partners (Waldby and Mitchell 2006; Landecker 2007). Advances in genomics and bioinformatics have since added complexity to the research situation, by increasing the chances that the genome of transformed donated tissue will at some point in time be sequenced, generating data that may concern not only the tissue provider but also her family, relatives and descendants.

This complexity has led to increasing concerns about the adequacy of current norms regulating research on human biological specimens. These norms were for the most part elaborated with the clinical trial as their basic model, in which the protection of the human subject means protection from being included in a research protocol without informed consent, particularly if such research involves an important departure from standard care and implies elevated risk of harm. The tendency has been to reason in terms of a subject who needs protection from bodily harm (as would be the case in clinical trials): if no such harm occurs in procuring residual tissue for research, then there should be no reason to require informed consent of the tissue provider. Until recently, less thought in terms of harm has been given to the possible impact for providers of the long-term separate existence of these specimens derived from their bodies and of the consequences that may ensue from the transformations these specimens undergo as a result of research practices. Even when the use of discarded tissue in research is requested explicitly – which is not always the case – the tissue provider may find it difficult to evaluate the meaning, purpose and ultimate value of donating discarded tissue, as well as the short- and long-term consequences of her act, for herself and for her family.

I would therefore like to consider the way in which the transformation of human biological materials into scientifically useful specimens and data through cell culturing, cryopreservation, and DNA sequencing poses specific challenges to the ethical norms that regulate tissue provision for research, and in particular, the norms of informed consent and respect for the provider's privacy. Indeed, because research on human tissue transforms the features and thus the initial value of these materials, often extending the possible consequences of this transformation in time and space, it becomes particularly difficult to define the conditions under which a provider's consent can be considered to be informed and the provider's identity and personal information protected.

To illustrate these difficulties, I will focus primarily, but not exclusively, on the use of surgically removed tissue that, in many treatment situations, is discarded. I will examine these issues from the perspective of a paradigm that has long been used in the analysis of practices involving the circulation of human biological materials: that of gift-giving. My principal example will be drawn from a case that dates back more than 50 years: the culturing of cervical tumour tissue that was excised during the course of treatment from a patient today known to be Henrietta Lacks and that ultimately gave rise to an immortal cell line known as HeLa. I would like to show how this and other examples raise basic issues that remain for the most part unresolved and that have become even more complex given contemporary scientific practices. All of these situations are characterized by research procedures that are initiated in the context of treatment and that tend to blur the usually more distinct boundaries between clinical situations and laboratory practices.

Discarded tissue and the gift relationship

In the early 1970s, three social scientists, one in the United Kingdom, and two in the United States, independently came up with the same idea: that an essay published in the 1920s by French sociologist and ethnographer Marcel Mauss entitled *Essai sur le Don* and translated into English as *The Gift*

(Mauss 1990 [1923–1924]) provided a pertinent conceptual framework for analysing the practices involved in the use of human body parts and substances for therapeutic purposes.

In the United Kingdom, Richard Titmuss, a specialist in social administration concerned with issues of welfare and social justice, wrote a book about the provision of blood for transfusion. His book entitled *The Gift Relationship* (Titmuss 1970) mobilizes Mauss' conceptual framework in comparing the way blood is procured in different societies. He concludes that systems relying on voluntary altruistic donation in the context of a public service are far superior in terms of their public health consequences than private commercial systems that rely on the selling of one's blood for a fee. Titmuss, basically concerned with the moral dimension of social policy issues, notably our collective regard or disregard for the needs of others (Titmuss 1970, 11), emphasized the gift's role in strengthening social ties and bringing about social cohesion, as developed by Mauss in his concluding chapters.

In the United States, sociologist Renée Fox with her colleague, historian Judith Swazey, applied Mauss' essay to a different field of therapeutic practices: the procurement and transplantation of vital body organs. They were initially made aware of the theme of the gift through its rhetorical use in medical and social policy discourse publicizing the need for organs (Fox 2011, 219); but as their field work developed, they realized that what they were observing had already been conceptualized by Mauss. Their book, *The Courage to Fail* (Fox and Swazey 1974), emphasizes the benefits of using the three-fold normative framework – involving the obligations to give, receive and give in return – that Mauss had identified as presiding over gift exchange to analyse the network of relationships that binds a live organ donor (usually a family member), the recipient and their kin. The ties binding these protagonists were in many ways "self-transcending" but they became at times mutually threatening – a phenomenon they termed the "tyranny of the gift" (Fox and Swazey 1974, 383). In their view, Mauss' framework had a limit in its application to this particular field: the organ as a gift is inherently impossible to reciprocate.

Much more could be said about each of these books and the insights each has brought as to the interest of using Mauss' essay in analysing practices involving the provision of body parts and substances for therapeutic purposes. Suffice it here to say that these three pioneers set a trend that has continued to this day: both Mauss' essay and the theme of the gift are constantly evoked in social science research on the donation of human biological materials, even if Mauss is sometimes only cited as a passing reference. The utility of the gift-exchange framework has since been questioned (Siminoff and Chillag 1999), although it is not clear if this critique is aimed at the rhetorical use of gift-giving or at the heuristic implications of Mauss' conceptual framework.

In the light of past applications and recent critiques of this framework, does it make sense to examine the use of residual human tissue for research from the perspective of the three-fold normative obligations conceptualized by Marcel Mauss in his essay on the gift in primitive societies (Mauss 1990

[1923–1924]; Novaes [Bateman] 1989)? Because discarded tissue is often perceived as valueless, framing the provision of discarded tissue for research purposes as a "gift" may initially seem inappropriate. However, Mauss emphasizes the fact that paradoxes are inherent to all objects circulating as gifts, and points to three of them.

The first is precisely that gifts are perceived as voluntary, disinterested and spontaneous forms of exchange. However, Mauss emphasizes that gift-giving is fundamentally an obligation because it is the expression of social ties, those ties that bind us to others: "To refuse to give, to fail to invite, just as to refuse to accept, is tantamount to declaring war; it is to reject the bond of alliance and commonality" (Mauss 1990, 13). This obligation is nonetheless experienced by the donor as something that is owed to the recipient and that is personally and fully assumed as such: "one gives because one is compelled to do so, because the recipient possesses some kind of right of property over anything that belongs to the donor. This ownership is expressed and conceived of as a spiritual bond" (Mauss 1990, 13). This "spiritual bond" between donor and recipient does not mean the recipient has a direct claim on the donor's gift: there is no right to expropriate or to pre-empt the donor's gesture. Giving must be voluntarily initiated by the donor.

The second crucial paradox is that objects exchanged within this framework are distinct from those exchanged in ordinary economic transactions between clans. They may have monetary value but, above all, they have subjective value because they are related to the donor's prestige and that of her clan, and as such can be considered as "part and parcel of his nature and substance", in other words, as a part of the donor's person. For this reason, objects exchanged within this framework cannot be appropriated by the recipient in the same way as in ordinary economic transactions: "To retain that thing would be dangerous and mortal, not only because it would be against the law and morality, but also because … the thing given is not inactive. Invested with life, often possessing individuality, it seeks to return to what [Robert] Hertz called its 'place of origin'" (Mauss 1990, 12–13).

Mauss thus emphasizes the problematic nature of putting such highly valued personal objects into circulation. Because they refer back to the person and the clan of the donor, they can never be totally dissociated from her, thus modulating the notion of the recipient's proprietary rights over the donor's gift mentioned above. Indeed, this strong "moral, physical and spiritual" attachment of the gift to the donor's own person and family obliges the recipient to treat the thing given in such a manner that it respects "the spiritual essence of the donor" contained in that thing. How this respect is put into practice has as much to do with the way the gift is received (and a gift cannot be received if it is not initially given) as it does with the way the gift is used or disposed of.

Moreover, because these objects are so personal, keeping them would be "dangerous", and "against the law and morality" (ibid.). Mauss therefore stresses – and this is our final element – the importance of giving something in return. However, he points out that returning a gift does not necessarily involve an immediate act that exonerates the recipient from her debt with regard to the donor; it more often involves a detour that implies passing the gift on to third parties not directly related to the initial donor, who in turn will themselves transfer back some other gift that they have received. In commenting on a text by Elsdon Best on exchange in Maori societies, Mauss notes that it is the very "spirit of the thing given" (the *hau*) that drives "all goods termed strictly personal" (*taonga*) along a circuit of deferred reciprocation. If one has been given such a good and then passed it on to a third party, "he gives another to me in turn, because he is impelled to do so by the *hau* my present possesses. I, for my part, am obliged to give you that thing because I must return to you what is in reality the effect of the *hau* of your *taonga*" (Mauss 1990, 11).

It is therefore not the transfer of ownership or the accumulation of property that is at stake in gift-giving as conceptualized by Mauss, but the capacity to maintain "alliance and commonality" through a constantly sustained movement of deferred reciprocity. Indeed, Mauss reminds us that "it is not individuals but collectivities that impose obligations of exchange and contract upon each other" (Mauss 1990, 5). His essay is thus not so much about individual gift-giving, as it is about maintaining a flow of voluntary transactions that constantly reinstate the ties guaranteeing group cohesion and ensuring fruitful and peaceful relationships with neighbouring groups.

Challenges to research ethics: a gift-giving perspective

Increased use of human biological materials for research has been accompanied by recurring revelations about breaches to good research practice, many of which concern the conditions in which tissue was provided for research. I contend that Mauss' three-fold normative framework on gift-giving can here be gainfully used as a heuristic tool to better understand the way in which these breaches undermine the network of relationships that sustain the transformation of human bodily materials into scientifically valuable specimens and possibly medically useful products.

Consent

The first and most obvious concern has been recurring breaches to the norm that requires *consent* from the provider. From a Maussian perspective, this is a crucial baseline condition if providing human tissue for research is to qualify as a gift. The highly publicized case of the HeLa cell line, derived from the biopsy of a cancer tumour excised from Henrietta Lacks in 1951 without her consent, popularized in a recent book by Rebecca Skloot, *The Immortal Life of Henrietta Lacks* (Skloot 2010), is one of many recent examples. There is also the well-known case of John Moore, whose spleen had been removed in 1976 as part of his treatment for hairy-cell cancer, but which was subsequently used without his consent to establish a lucrative cell line named MO (later renamed RLC) (Waldby 2006, ch. 3; Truog *et al.* 2012). These cases point to the fact that discarded tissue has almost always been used without obtaining explicit consent from the person who provided the material, unless obtaining the material requires a medical procedure unnecessary to standard care. In Moore's case, even this latter precaution was not respected, as it would seem that in recommending surgery, Moore's physician was conscious of the fact that "Moore's diseased cells produced large amounts of lymphokines … [and that these proteins were] of use and interest to many researchers" (Waldby and Mitchell 2006, 88).

Concerning the case of Henrietta Lacks, whether or not there was a breach to the norm of consent is an open question. The cell line was established in 1951, two years after the redaction of the Nuremberg Code, based on memoranda established in view of the Doctor's Trial as a basis for the indictment and prosecution of the defendants. The Nuremberg Code states as its first and most important principle: "The voluntary consent of the human subject is absolutely essential". This principle was already part of probably the first known code of research ethics, *Principles of Ethics Concerning Experimentation with Human Beings*, established in 1946, just after the Second World War by the American Medical Association (Shuster 1997). The principle of voluntary consent was therefore not unknown at the time that Henrietta Lacks was a patient, which does not mean it was well-known or applied.

The principle was reiterated in greater detail in a document prepared in 1953 by the National Institutes of Health (NIH) for its Clinical Center Policy, most of which is devoted to the "Group Consideration of Clinical Research Procedures Deviating from Accepted Medical Practice or Involving Unusual Hazard". Numerous excerpts from its section III, *Principals* [sic] *Governing Physician–Patient Relationship*, resonate with contemporary ethical norms for consent in human subject research:

> 2 Information for Patient
>
> … Each prospective patient will be given an oral explanation in terms suited to his comprehension, supplemented by general written information or other appropriate means, of his role as a patient in the Clinical Center, the nature of the proposed investigation and particularly any potential danger to him.
>
> 3 Patient Understanding and Agreement
>
> (a). Standard consent or agreement forms shall be used for surgery, anaesthesia, photography and other procedures where they are ordinarily required and for permission to disclose clinical findings, records, or other personal information …
>
> (c). … When … a procedure involves an unusual hazard, the proposed procedure shall not be undertaken until the patient has voluntarily signed a statement, entered on the patient's chart or as a separate

> memorandum, indicating his understanding of the procedure and its purpose, including potential hazards to him, and his willingness to participate.
>
> (NIH 1953, 5)

However, the notion of "clinical research procedures deviating from accepted medical practice or involving unusual hazard" suggests that these elaborate norms of consent applied only to situations in which there was a risk of direct harm to the patient. This is exemplified by a paragraph in the policy defining such hazards:

> Two distinct types of hazard are recognized: (a) jeopardy to the life or relative state of well-being of the research subject ...; (b) jeopardy to the subject's chances for cure of his illness or alleviation of his symptoms, occasioned by withholding or delaying the application of established therapeutic procedures.
>
> (ibid., 3)

Thus, although the principle of consent was an established deontological norm since at least 1946, it is not clear that this norm was enforceable or even applied to procedures that involved no extra risk or intervention for a patient. Institutional oversight of "investigations involving human beings, including clinical research" was instated a bit later, in 1966, when the Surgeon General's Directives (Office of the Surgeon General 1967, 350) pointed out "the need for group review to protect the rights and welfare of the human subjects involved".

Ambiguity about consent with respect to the collection of discarded tissue remains even today, as illustrated by the following excerpt from the present US Code of Federal Regulations – *US 45 CFR 46: Subtitle A – Basic HHS Policy for Protection of Human Subjects*: Sec §46.101 – for the most part established in 1991:

> (b) ... are exempt from this policy:
>
> (4) Research involving the collection or study of existing data, documents, records, pathological specimens or diagnostic specimens if these sources are publicly available *or* if the information is recorded by the investigator in such a manner that subjects cannot be identified, directly or through identifiers linked to the subjects.
>
> (p. 104 – my emphasis)

Given mounting concern about appropriate oversight for research on human biological specimens, the Office for Human Research Protection (OHRP) and the Department of Health and Human Services (HHS) have since proposed a set of recommendations for research involving "coded private information or biological specimens" (OHRP and HHS 2008) that would further limit exemptions from research oversight to situations that meet not one or the other, but both of the conditions mentioned above. In other words, only specimens from publicly available collections (thus not involving direct interactions between a researcher and the tissue providers) and only those specimens that are not identifiable should be exempt from research oversight. All other situations should be subjected to IRB review, as specified by the Code of Federal Regulations. So far, these recommendations have not been transposed into government policy (OHRP and HHS 2008, 3–4; Bledsoe and Grizzle 2013; *Nature* 2013a).

In other words, were the Henrietta Lacks case to occur today, the physician who excises the tissue for research purposes and the researcher who uses it to establish a cell line would be exempt from research oversight, if their research were able to meet the second condition of 45 CFR 46.101–2. 4, that is, if the specimen obtained and the information associated with it could be totally de-identified. Why is this so, despite an abundant literature and increasing concern about breaches in ethical norms? There are indications that a competing concern exists among professionals who fear that a tightening of restrictions may lead to an eventual "shortage" of available material for research – a term often heard in relation to the procurement of organs for transplantation. Indeed, a recent editorial in *Nature* commenting on a Welsh proposal to introduce presumed consent for the procurement of tissue after death, goes so far as to suggest that presumed consent, if too radical a solution as yet, might one day be a reasonable option:

> Presumed consent, with the burden placed on people and families to opt-out of tissue donation, seems a step too far *at present* for material needed for scientific research. But are the issues involved that different from those surrounding transplantation? Both promise better health and new life from the waste of death.
>
> (*Nature* 2013b, 6 – my emphasis)

Because this comment is made in the context of "a time of increasing scrutiny of the way in which tissue taken during hospital procedures is used in medical and scientific research" (*Nature* 2013b, 6), it seems likely that presumed consent may also be seen by the author of the editorial as an acceptable option for tissue provision more generally. From the point of view of Mauss' essay, a policy of presumed consent, applied strictly, would imply a decision to withdraw tissue provision from a gift-giving normative framework, because it pre-empts the opportunity of the donor or her family to have an active voice in this system of reciprocal obligations.

Informed consent

A second reason for concern is related to the increasing number of collections of cryopreserved human biological specimens. Many of these collections are established in connection with a specific research project, although very often the samples will be used again for new projects. Some collections known as "biobanks" or "biorepositories" have been created independently of any immediately identifiable research project, in order to make tissue specimens generally available to researchers over a considerable length of time. As we have already seen above, de-identified samples from these collections also offer the advantage of exempting the researcher from having to undergo oversight procedures. However, the existence of these collections implies a wider variety of possible uses of donated human specimens, thus increasing the complexity of the situations that will have to be explained to donors – whether these are patients or healthy volunteers. In other words, collections generate unprecedented questions *about how informed a tissue provider's consent really is* – put in Maussian terms, how clearly the donor perceives the network of relationships being served by her gift.

If we return to the case of Henrietta Lacks, she of course was informed of nothing since her consent had not been sought. However, members of her family were solicited on several occasions to give their consent for various procedures related to the existence of the HeLa cells. Exchanges with the physicians and researchers they met on these occasions illustrate the potential for misunderstanding and conflict ensuing from these situations.

The first occasion arose just after Henrietta Lack's death when George Gey, the researcher who had cultured the tissue from her tumour, wanted samples from as many other organs as possible in her body to see if they would grow like the cells cultured from her tumour (they didn't). Permission for an autopsy was therefore requested of Henrietta's husband, David Lacks (also known as Day); however, when he was first asked – by telephone, when he was also told of his wife's death, he said no. However when he later went to the hospital, with a cousin, to see Henrietta's body and deal with the ensuing paperwork, the physicians once again asked for permission to perform an autopsy: "They said they wanted *to run tests that might help his children someday.* Day's cousin said *it wouldn't hurt*, so eventually Day agreed and signed an autopsy permission form" (Skloot 2010, 89–90 – my emphasis). Skloot makes no comment as to what David Lacks had understood as regards "tests that might help his children someday". The cousin's remark suggests an autopsy would not harm them.

More than 20 years later, in 1973, researchers again became interested in contacting Henrietta's Lacks' family, because the research community had discovered that the HeLa cell line had most probably contaminated the cell cultures most commonly used by researchers world-wide. Indeed, they had discovered that the cultures all contained a rare genetic marker called glucose-6-phosphate dehydrogenase-A (G6PD-A), present almost exclusively in black Americans. By contacting the family and drawing blood from several family members, they hoped to be able to develop genetic tests that might help them identify a genetic marker specific to the HeLa cells in culture (ibid., 152–157).

There are several accounts of what happened. Skloot relates that the family did agree to have their blood drawn, but that there was a misunderstanding concerning the reason for drawing blood. Her account of one such event involves Susan Hsu, a post-doctoral fellow working with Victor McKusick, the leading geneticist at Johns Hopkins where Henrietta Lacks had been treated. After Hsu had called to make an appointment to go to Day's home to draw blood, Day "called [his children] Lawrence, Sonny and Deborah, saying 'You got to come over to the house tomorrow, *doctors from Hopkins coming to test everybody's blood to see if you all got that cancer your mother had*'". Several days after Hsu and a colleague from McKusick's lab had come by to draw blood, Day's daughter Deborah "called Hopkins again and again telling the switchboard operators, '*I'm calling for my cancer results.*' But none of the operators knew what tests she was talking about, or where to send her for help" (ibid., 184, 185 – my emphasis).

When Skloot interviewed Victor McKusick and Susan Hsu, she asked them about this misunderstanding. McKusick responded: "I suspect there was no effort to explain anything in great detail. But I don't believe anyone would have told them we were testing for cancer because that was not the case" (ibid., 183). As for Susan Hsu, she was shocked to learn that there had been a misunderstanding: "'I feel very bad', she said. 'People should have told them. You know, we never thought at that time they did not understand'" (ibid., 189). Hsu had obviously forgotten that she was one of the persons who had come to draw the blood, and was therefore one of the "people who should have told them".

Another account involves a person who at the time was also a research fellow at McKusick's lab: the British medical geneticist Peter Harper. This account is given in the context of a review of Rebecca Skloot's book, written by Harper himself and published in *Human Genetics* in 2011. Harper describes a first contact with the Lacks family in 1971 that apparently predates the incident related above. His attempt to locate the family and subsequent encounter with the family, as he recalls it in his review article, gives us a further view into the difficulty researchers experience in communicating their needs to persons who have lost a family member to cancer. Indeed, to Harper's surprise, the Lacks seemed quite ready and willing to let him not only draw blood but also take a small skin pinch biopsy for culturing fibroblasts; but he admits to not having provided them with any explanation as to why he wished to collect these tissue samples: "What did I tell them about the reason? *I do not think that I could have given any real information of help to them nor did they ask me. I certainly did not get written consent*" (Harper 2011, 464 – my emphasis). The Lacks family's willingness to cooperate left a strong and lasting impression on Harper: "the 1971 episode remained in my memory, and still does as *an example of how ordinary people were prepared to be trusting and altruistic in a situation where there was no clear benefit to them*" (ibid. – my emphasis). However, in view of the lack of information they had as to the purpose of his request to draw blood and take skin cells, the Lacks were indeed trusting, but maybe not altruistic in that they were under the misguided impression that some direct clinical benefit could be expected from what they seem to have perceived as blood tests.

Several more recent cases equally illustrate how the collection and use of human biological specimens and associated clinical data create potential for misunderstanding and conflict between researchers and providers of human tissue. The first is a well-known lawsuit filed by the Havasupai tribe against the researchers from Arizona State University, who had used far more widely and without specific consent, the biological specimens initially provided by members of the tribe for research on diabetes.[1] Whereas the researchers seem to have provided consent forms addressing the issue of future use of the collected samples – what is known as broad consent – oral exchanges between researchers and the tribe were focused on diabetes, the tribe's more immediate health concern. Thus, even if the researchers' paperwork may have been in order from a strictly legal point of view, they failed to establish the necessary transparency and trust with regard to the tissue providers that would have allowed them to continue the research they had initiated. The lawsuit resulted in a large out of court settlement in 2010 and the destruction of all the collected samples (McEwen *et al.* 2013, 379).

Another recent case shows how easily the borders between clinical care and research are crossed. A lawsuit was filed in 2009 against the state of Texas by parents who realized that dried blood spots, resulting from the mandatory newborn screening of their children, were being collected and used for research purposes without parental consent and more generally, without public awareness that research was being conducted on these samples. As in the preceding case, the settlement of the lawsuit resulted in the destruction of samples, as no justification and thus no consecutive authorization had been given to store them (McEwen *et al.* 2013, 378).

In all of these cases, there had been initial consent to provide biological specimens (and in the case of the parents, adherence or at least compliance to mandatory screening), but the providers had not fully understood what was going to be done with the materials and data they had consented to give, nor whose purposes were being served. Collecting human materials for research in a context where multiple research projects may ultimately be served by the existence of these specimens is far more difficult to explain to providers than the request for a vital organ in view of the therapeutic needs of an anonymous patient.

Ethicists have tried to address this difficulty by elaborating new paradigms for informed consent. Blanket consents imply unconditional acceptance of all possible uses of provided samples. Broad consent involves consenting to research that is conducted within a certain framework, and may imply, in case of a change of framework, the possibility of re-consent. Both of these models imply a more passive form of consent, in which decision-making about the appropriate use of samples is left to the researcher under conditions established in the consent form. Dynamic consent, on the other hand, implies greater interaction between donors and researchers, often through internet technology, giving the donor a more active, durable control over the use of her samples (Meslin and Cho 2010; Steinsbekk *et al.* 2013; *Nature* 2013c; McEwen *et al.* 2013).

There is no consensus in the research or the bioethical milieu as to which paradigm is best adapted to present research situations; and not all potential tissue providers will have the same needs and expectations as to how they wish their tissue samples to be used. Moreover, the simple fact that some "immortal" cell lines, cryopreserved specimens and dematerialized data can theoretically be stored indefinitely, even after the death of tissue providers, tempers any expectations that a provider can be truly informed of all possible uses of donated samples.

The solution to this difficulty is far from evident and may lie, not as much in finding the most appropriate legal paradigm for fully informed consent, as in creating the conditions for improved transparency in the relationship between donor and recipient. For indeed, consent that is not appropriately informed is equivalent to no consent at all: as the examples above so explicitly show, human tissue unknowingly provided for research is considered by providers as taken rather than as given. Indeed, from a Maussian perspective, the donor has been misled as to the network of relationships that her gift serves. Greater fiduciary responsibility of the recipient in requesting and handling research tissue, without excluding appropriate oversight and sanctions for overt misuse of tissue samples, but also greater citizen awareness of what is going on both in medical research and in science, may be the only way to increase non-naïve and non-exploitative participation in the scientific enterprise.

Protection of privacy

The collection of human research specimens also implies the collection of large quantities of personal and health data, often in dematerialized forms. This has generated increasing unease as to the research community's capacity to *protect the privacy* of research participants. This concern has now been magnified by the fact that many tissue samples have been subjected to the potent tools of next generation sequencing and bioinformatics analysis, generating quantities of genomic data that is shared in public databases by scientists world-wide. Indeed, genomics researchers share an unprecedented amount of data, as illustrated by the creation, in June 2013, of a Global Alliance assembling more than 150 research institutions world-wide for the responsible sharing of genomic and clinical data.

The sequencing of the HeLa cell more than 60 years after the cell line was created (EMBL 2013) illustrates the difficulty of protecting the privacy of the tissue provider and her family in the age of genomics. However, this breach to Henrietta Lacks' privacy was made possible by an earlier breach to her privacy in 1971.

In 1970, Howard Jones, the Johns Hopkins gynaecologist who had treated Henrietta Lacks, decided to publish an article on the history of the HeLa cell line as a tribute to George Gey who had just died (Jones et al. 1971; Skloot 2010, 172; Harper 2011, 464). Until 1971, all the persons involved in the establishment of the cell line had kept the provider's identity secret. But given the "immortality" of the cell line – it is proliferating even today – there had already been much speculation as to who the tissue provider had been. When Jones consulted the medical file to prepare the article, he discovered not only photographs of the original biopsy, but also a copy of a photograph of Henrietta Lacks, which according to Peter Harper, was lent by David Lacks (Harper 2011, 464). Given that 20 years had elapsed, Jones felt it would be acceptable to reveal both the name of the person whose tumour tissue had been at the origin of the HeLa cell and publish her photograph; the publication also revealed elements of her medical history that helped explain why the tissue had proliferated as it did. As Skloot puts it, this revelation would "forever [link] Henrietta, Lawrence, Sonny, Deborah, Zakariyya, their children, and all future generations of Lackses to the HeLa cells, and the DNA inside them" (Skloot 2010, 173).

The second breach to her privacy simply magnifies the effects of the first. In 2013, a group of German researchers sequenced the HeLa cell and, as is today the norm in good scientific practice, made the data freely available to researchers all over the world (EMBL 2013). Henrietta's Lacks' family immediately challenged this, saying that the data also made publicly available information that might directly concern their own health as her descendants. The data were immediately withdrawn, and ultimately an agreement was reached between the family and the National Institutes of Health: all genomic data derived from the HeLa cell must be deposited in a controlled access database, with requests for access to data requiring review by a six-member panel, of which two members are her descendants. The National Institutes of Health said it would enforce adherence to this agreement by all researchers using federal funds, but quite obviously, it will be unable to enforce such a practice among researchers funded with private funds or located anywhere else in the world than in the United States (Hudson and Collins 2013; Callaway 2013).

Indeed, despite legislation in many countries protecting the privacy of genetic data, there is a risk that data may be accessed by unauthorized persons. In May 2013, Yaniv Erlich, a computational biologist presently working at the Whitehead Institute for Biomedical Research in Cambridge, Massachusetts, and his doctoral student Melissa Gymrek demonstrated, by using Y chromosome short tandem repeats (STR) as markers, that the identity of anonymous research participants can be easily ascertained through the cross-referencing of anonymous research sample data with genetic information publicly available online through social media posts and entries on genealogy websites (Hayden 2013; Gymrek *et al.* 2013).[2] This has led to technical measures intended to better ensure the privacy of personal data, such as creating different levels of access to data: aggregate, non-identified data is left in open access public databases, while individual data with identifiers are stored in controlled access databases. Nonetheless, a significant part of the problem, as demonstrated by Gymrek's and Erlich's experiment, are the large quantities of personal and health data already made freely available online by private individuals.

For this reason, some have suggested that increasing protective measures for personal and genomic data in the digital age is useless: on the contrary, data should be shared openly and voluntarily in the public domain. Geneticist George Church founded the Personal Genome Project in 2005 precisely on that premise, but he requires volunteers to undergo an "entrance exam" that ensures they have an understanding of genetics and are informed of the risks of participation (for example, discrimination linked to disability or disease, but also possible use of their DNA without their consent, etc.) (McEwen *et al.* 2013, 378; Sun 2014). In other words, they are warned that by sharing genomic and personal data, they will encounter the same issues and concerns, including potential for misuse of their data, raised by the circulation of genomic data in more standard frameworks.

Genetic and genomic research have also raised unprecedented questions about the occasional desirability of re-identifying tissue providers when research uncovers "incidental findings", that is, information that may be clinically actionable or otherwise personally useful (McEwen et al. 2013; van Veen 2013). Should anonymous research participants, who would normally no longer be solicited after providing a sample, be advised if a mutation, such as the BRCA gene, associated with hereditary breast and ovarian cancer, turns up in the results of research unrelated to this condition? How should such situations be handled? Should participants be asked in advance whether or not they wish to be contacted in such cases? Is this a decision that should be left to them or to the physician–investigator conducting the research? Can this treatment benefit from unexpected research findings be considered a form of reciprocation? These issues call into question once again the supposedly impermeable boundaries between research and treatment.

It is notable that both John Moore and the descendants of Henrietta Lacks were first alerted to the creation of a cell line from their or their ascendant's tissue by the fact that researchers had contacted them again to draw blood. Re-establishing contact with a research participant is therefore a moment in which any irregularity arising within the gift-giving framework will come to the fore. In John Moore's case, he became aware of the value that his tissue had acquired after transformation by the researchers, but he also became aware of the fact that researchers were trying to keep him from finding out what benefits had accrued from this value. In the case of Henrietta Lacks' descendants, not only was there confusion as to the purpose for drawing blood from the family, since they had mistakenly understood there would be an immediate clinical benefit for them; they also became progressively aware of the fact that whatever clinical application might eventually be derived from research with the HeLa cells, it would never benefit them, because their limited financial resources excluded them de facto from the health system in which the return on the research investment is made. In other words, their gift served a network of relationships in which the flow of transactions ultimately eluded them.

Conclusion

In the light of this brief overview of the way in which the present use of residual tissue for research challenges the ethical norms of informed consent and respect for the provider's privacy, Mauss' conceptualization of the three-fold normative framework that binds protagonists involved in gift exchange can be considered, within limits, as a pertinent heuristic tool in examining the relationships set up around the provision, transformation and use of discarded tissue for research. It directs our attention to a basic requirement for consent that must be appropriately informed, if tissue provision is to fit the norm of a "thing given" rather than taken. It also points to the fact that the non-conflictual circulation of "gifts" is better served by a network of relationships with clearly identifiable parties and objectives. The transparency of the network and of its objectives tends to disappear as the borders distinguishing different areas of activity, such as medical care and research, are blurred. This is especially true when the "gift" may ultimately be of unlimited use to multiple unidentifiable partners over time. As one loses sight of the network within which gifts circulate and are disposed of, there is a corresponding loss of trust and potential for conflict among protagonists in the network.

The threefold normative framework that binds the protagonists of such a network – giving, receiving, returning – encounters its limits when confronted with the fact that research is conducted within a competing framework where scientific careers and industrial interests are at stake; there is an evident tension, although not necessarily an incompatibility, between the norms and values that are specific to the research framework and those that apply to the gift-giving framework. As long as gift-giving is considered a pertinent framework for understanding the circulation of human biological materials – which may not be the case in the future – this framework suggests that scientific, professional and financial incentives must never override the legitimate interests and rights of the tissue providers who have agreed to put highly personal material and data into the hands of researchers. The respect for these rights and interests seems to depend, in my reading of Mauss' essay on the gift, on the constant flow of "life-giving" substances through a circuit of deferred reciprocation in which the "spirit of the thing given" remains constantly present in research activity, the benefits of which should ultimately find their way back to the community that initiated the giving. For, precisely, Mauss' essay is not about reciprocation in the sense of immediate compensation or benefit to the initial donor: it is about the constant effort to maintain social cohesion in our search for improved solutions to collective problems that must ultimately benefit all.

Acknowledgements

Work for this article was supported by the SIRIC programme of the Institut Curie (Paris, France).

Notes

1 See http://genetics.ncai.org/case-study/havasupai-Tribe.cfm.
2 Genetic genealogy databases make available information that links Y chromosome short tandem repeats (STR) to particular surnames.

References

Bledsoe, M.J., and W.E. Grizzle. 2013. "Use of Human Specimens in Research: The Evolving United States Regulatory, Policy and Scientific Landscape." *Diagnostic Histopathology* 13(3): 322–330.

Callaway, E. 2013. "Deal Done over HeLa Cell Line." *Nature* 500, 8 August: 132–133.

EMBL (European Molecular Biology Laboratory). 2013. Press Release: *Havoc in Biology's Most-used Human Cell Line: Genome of HeLa Cells Sequenced for the First Time*. Heidelberg, 11 March. Available at: www.embl.de/aboutus/communication_outreach/media_relations/2013/130311_Heidelberg/PR_Steinmetz_Havoc_in_biologys_mostused_human_cell_line.pdf.

Fox, R.C. 2011. *In the Field: A Sociologist's Journey*. New Brunswick, NJ: Transaction Publishers.

Fox, R.C., and J.P. Swazey. 1974. *The Courage to Fail: A Social View of Organ Transplants and Dialysis*. Chicago: University of Chicago Press.

Global Alliance. 2013. Creating a Global Alliance to Enable Responsible Sharing of Genomic and Clinical Data. Broad Institute, June 3. Available at: www.broadinstitute.org/files/news/pdfs/GAWhitePaperJune3.pdf.

Gymrek, M., McGuire, A.L., Golan, D., Halperin, E., and Y. Erlich. 2013. "Identifying Personal Genomes by Surname Inference." *Science* 339: 321–324.

Harper, P.S. 2011. "Book Review – Rebecca Skloot: The Immortal Life of Henrietta Lacks." *Human Genetics* 129: 463–464.

Hayden, E.C. 2013. "The Genome Hacker." *Nature* 497, 9 May: 172–174.

Hudson, K.L., and F.S. Collins. 2013. "Family Matters." *Nature* 500, 8 August: 143–144.

Jones Jr, H.W., McKusick, V.A., Harper, P.S., and K.D. Wuu. 1971. "George Otto Gey, 1899–1970. The HeLa Cell and a Reappraisal of Its Origin." *Obstetrics and Gynecology* 38, 6 December: 945–949.

Landecker, H. 2007. *Culturing Life: How Cells Became Technologies*. Cambridge, MA: Harvard University Press.

Mauss, M. 1990 [1923–1924]. *The Gift: The Form and Reason for Exchange in Archaic Societies*. Translated by W.D. Halls, foreword by M. Douglas. New York: W.W. Norton and Co.

McEwen, J.E., Boyer, J.T., and K.Y. Sun. 2013. "Evolving Approaches to the Ethical Management of Genomic Data." *Trends in Genetics* 29(6): 375–381.

Meslin, E.M., and M.K. Cho. 2010. "Research Ethics in the Era of Personalized Medicine: Updating Science's Contract with Society." *Public Health Genomics* 13: 378–384.

Nature. 2013a. Editorial. "A Culture of Consent." *Nature* 498, 27 June: 407.

Nature. 2013b. Editorial. "Presumed Consent." *Nature* 499, 4 July: 6.

Nature. 2013c. Editorial. "Blood Ties." *Nature* 500, 8 August: 121.

NIH (National Institutes of Health). 1953. *Medical Board Document no. 1: Organization, Functions and Authority of the Medical Board of the Clinical Center*. Available at: http://history.nih.gov/research/downloads/NIH1953humansubjectpolicy.pdf.

Novaes [Bateman], S.B. 1989. "Giving, Receiving, Repaying: Gamete Donors and Donor Policies in Reproductive Medicine." *International Journal for Technology Assessment in Health Care* 5(4): 639–657.

Office of the Surgeon General, US Public Health Service. 1967 [1966]. "The Surgeon General's Directives on Human Experimentation." *American Psychologist* 22(5): 350–355.

OHRP and HHS (Office for Human Research Protections and Department of Health and Human Services). 2008. Guidance on Research Involving Coded Private Information or Biological Specimens. Available at: www.hhs.gov/ohrp/policy/cdebiol.html.

Shuster, E. 1997. "Fifty Years Later: The Significance of the Nuremberg Code." *New England Journal of Medicine* 337(20): 1436–1440.

Siminoff, L.A., and K. Chillag. 1999. "The Fallacy of the 'Gift of Life'." *Hastings Center Report* 29(6): 34–41.

Skloot, R. 2010. *The Immortal Life of Henrietta Lacks*. New York: Crown Publishers.

Steinsbekk, K.S., Myskja, B.K., and B. Solberg. 2013. "Broad Consent versus Dynamic Consent in Biobank Research: Is Passive Participation an Ethical Problem?" *European Journal of Human Genetics* 21: 897–902.

Sun, A. 2014. "For Volunteers, a DNA Database." *New York Times*, April 28. Available at: www.nytimes.com/2014/04/29/science/from-volunteers-a-dna-database.html?emc=edit_tnt_20140428&nlid=17076778&tntemail0=y.

Titmuss, R.M. 1970. *The Gift Relationship: From Human Blood to Social Policy*. London: George Allen & Unwin Ltd.

Truog, R.D., Kesselheim, A.S., and S. Joffe. 2012. "Paying Patients for Their Tissue: The Legacy of Henrietta Lacks." *Science* 337, 6 July: 37–38.

van Veen, E.-B. 2013. "Europe and Tissue Research: A Regulatory Patchwork." *Diagnostic Histopathology* 19(9): 331–336.

Waldby, C., and R. Mitchell. 2006. *Tissue Economies: Blood, Organs, and Cell Lines in Late Capitalism*. Durham and London: Duke University Press.

4 "I wouldn't put them on eBay!"

Discourses on money, markets and meanings amongst IVF patients volunteering for a UK "egg sharing for research" scheme

Erica Haimes

Introduction

The growing global demand for human tissue for research and treatment is accompanied by debates about ethically appropriate ways of encouraging individuals to donate tissue (Nuffield Council on Bioethics 2011). These include debates about the ethics of offering money "for", or in association with, the provision of tissue. Concerns include whether offers of money: constitute an undue inducement; compromise individual autonomy and the ability to give informed consent; exploit poorer populations; contribute to the commodification of the human body; compromise human dignity; crowd out other values such as altruism (Radin 1996; Svenaeus 2010; Nuffield Council on Bioethics 2011; Sandel 2012; Hoeyer 2013).

Particular concerns have been raised about offering money to women to encourage them to provide eggs and other reproductive tissue for research (Braun and Schulz 2012; Roxland 2012; Haimes *et al.* 2013). For example, should women undergoing IVF have to consider the loss of their eggs to research when they might need them for treatment (Waldby and Carroll 2012), and should non-IVF patients undergo the potential physical risks of IVF when there is no therapeutic need for them to do so (HFEA 2006)?

However, these debates lack insight from the very populations under discussion: those who provide tissue. To rectify that deficit this chapter draws on a socio-ethical investigation of the views and experiences of women who have volunteered for a UK scheme providing eggs for research. This scheme, which I shall refer to as the "Newcastle Egg Sharing for Research scheme" (the NESR) is considered controversial because it advertises for current IVF patients to "share" 50% of the eggs they produce in a single IVF cycle (as long as they produce six or more eggs); those who provide eggs receive a £1,500 discount on their private IVF fees for that cycle (currently £3,000–£3,700). The eggs provided go towards somatic cell nuclear transfer research and, more recently, to research on avoiding the transmission of mitochondrial diseases.

A brief overview of international legislation and regulation

One reason why the NESR is considered controversial (either progressive or transgressive) and has attracted criticism (Waldby *et al.* 2013) is that it appears not to conform to European legislation or practice (Braun and Schulz 2012). However, although the EU appears to place clear restrictions on the offer of incentives for the donation of body parts, the Nuffield Council on Bioethics (2011) draws attention to the varying ways in which the potential entanglements of money and human tissue are actually described. While some EU documents insist that donation should be "unpaid", and procurement be on a "non-profit basis", the Oviedo Convention states that the human body and its parts "shall not, as such, give rise to financial gain" (cited in Nuffield Council on Bioethics 2011, 70). The "as such" remains unexplicated (Pattinson 2012). The World Health Organization bans "monetary payments" or "rewards" and the Declaration of Istanbul calls for a ban on organs being "bought or sold for material gain". The UK Human Tissue Act distinguishes between "commercial dealings", "rewards" (financial or material) and "reimbursements" in the supply of human material (Nuffield Council on Bioethics 2011, 70).

The researcher-clinicians who designed the NESR were licensed to implement it by the Human Fertilisation and Embryology Authority (HFEA) in 2007. They claimed, amidst controversy, that the NESR mirrored the well-established "egg sharing" for treatment scheme, in which one infertile woman pays for the treatment of another infertile woman when receiving half her eggs. Roberts and Throsby (2008, 161) argued this claim was a way of establishing the NESR as "business as usual", silencing ethical objections. Since October 2011, the HFEA has allowed payments, for expenses and inconvenience, of £750 per cycle for egg donors and £35 per visit for sperm donors (Hamm and Anton 2012). These amounts were designed to encourage donation for treatment and research, without "attracting those who are merely financially motivated" (Pattinson 2012, 583).

In the USA practice is varied. Since 2009, New York State's stem cell board allow "compensation", beyond direct expenses, to women who provide their eggs for research: up to US$5,000 is considered reasonable; US$5,000 to US $10,000 requires further justification, and amounts over US$10,000 are prohibited (Roxland 2012; Haimes *et al.* 2013, 285). Egli *et al.* (2011) concluded that American women elsewhere who had volunteered, but failed to proceed, to donate eggs for research did so because they were not offered financial compensation. Noggle *et al.* (2011) offered financial compensation to American women volunteering to provide eggs for either treatment or research and reported that some did donate to research. Neither article reported any systematic investigation or analysis of the women's reasoning. Clearly there are different views over the desirable relationship between money and body parts and over the ways in which that relationship can, and should, be characterized (Svenaeus 2010).

Characterizing the debate on money and bodies

A brief overview of the debates can be gained by comparing two prominent accounts: Sandel (2012) and the Nuffield Council on Bioethics (2011) report. There are many other participants in these debates as the references cited hitherto indicate; I have chosen these simply because they "represent" different conclusions, while exploring similar terrain.

Sandel (2012, 8) "represents" the concerns raised over the moral implications of the progressive monetization of social life, suggesting that this increases both inequality and corruption. He argues that when everything can be bought and sold, those with less money are excluded from full social participation, and that market values corrupt or "crowd out" other, more important, values (ibid., 9). Attaching a price to the "good things in life" makes them worth more, financially, but degrades how we value them because our attitudes to them change. He is concerned that we will devalue human beings if we treat them or their body parts as commodities to be bought and sold for profit. These are moral and political issues: "To resolve them we have to debate, case by case, the moral meaning of these goods and the proper way of valuing them" (ibid., 10).

Finding a resolution is complicated by having to decide whether to participate in "morally questionable markets" in order to achieve desirable ends, such as having children (ibid., 79) or, perhaps, advancing clinical research. Will marketizing such practices by, for example, introducing incentives, "displace" non-market norms (ibid., 90)? Instead of focusing on whether particular incentives will "work" (e.g. "Will researchers recruit more egg donors by providing incentives to donate?") a moral assessment should be made "of the attitudes and norms that money may … crowd out", in case this changes "the character of the activity in ways we would (or at least should) regret? If so, should we avoid introducing financial incentives into the activity, even though they might do some good?" (ibid., 91). He acknowledges that some exchanges can appear to benefit both parties without anyone else suffering but is concerned that such exchanges can nonetheless diminish the value of that which is being exchanged; those goods become tainted by the very fact of exchange (ibid., 114). Sandel's worry is that "the marketization of everything" diminishes shared citizenship, so those with money, and those without, lead increasingly separate lives (ibid., 203).

In contrast to Sandel, the Nuffield Council on Bioethics noted that while they value the altruistic donation of human material they do not accept that systems based on altruism and systems involving payment are "necessarily incompatible" (Nuffield Council on Bioethics 2011, viii). They reject Sandel's "crowding out" argument and do not regard the offer of money as necessarily unethical. They suggest, however, that the following require close scrutiny when money is offered: the welfare of the donor; the welfare of "closely concerned" individuals; the potential threat to the common good, and the professional responsibilities of the health practitioners (ibid., 7–8). This contention that money is not inherently contaminating is important, in light of the reference to "gifts" as "the sanctioned metaphor" for bodily contributions (Svenaeus 2010).

As we have seen, the Nuffield Council on Bioethics identify different ways in which the use of money is described, so they propose their own typology. All transactions involving money should be termed "payments" and different types of payments then distinguished as follows: (i) "recompense" for losses incurred (as "reimbursement" of expenses or "compensation" for non-financial losses); (ii) "rewards" that constitute a material advantage for donating, which could include "remuneration" if wage-based, and (iii) "purchase", defined as "payment in direct exchange for something (e.g. a certain amount for a kidney, or per egg)" (Nuffield Council on Bioethics 2011, 70).

The report adopts an "intervention ladder" through which the ethical acceptability of any intervention to encourage donation might be evaluated. Rung 1 interventions would just be information about donating; rung 6, the highest, would include financial incentives that leave the donor financially better off as a result of donating (ibid., viii–ix). Rung 6 interventions are no less ethical than rung 1 but their ethical implications require closer scrutiny because of their potential threat "to wider communal values" (ibid., 5). The authors also distinguish between "altruist-focused" and "non-altruist focused interventions" where the former are intended to remove barriers to people who are "already inclined to donate" and the latter intended to encourage donation by offering a reward "sufficient to prompt action" (ibid., 5). They "reject the concept of the purchase of bodily material, where money exchanges hands in direct return for body parts" and distinguish "purchase" from uses of money that "reward or recompense donors" (ibid., 5). The amount of "work" that this report needs to do, to build an argument for allowing money to be involved, is noteworthy, underscoring the assumption in most debates that the entanglement of money and body parts is damaging.

Despite their differences, the Nuffield Council on Bioethics and Sandel agree on the need to attend to the detail of particular cases and contexts. Sandel (2012, 10) calls for a "case by case" debate and the Chair of the Nuffield Council on Bioethics says, "this enquiry has enabled us to *compare* how particular ethical ideas and concepts are used in different circumstances, and has thus helped us understand the importance of the *context* in which decisions and actions take place" (Nuffield Council on Bioethics 2011, viii; emphasis in original). Nonetheless, each relies on claims about the motives and preferences of the people directly involved in these areas. I want to ask instead how those directly involved characterize their own motivations, preferences and actions. In order to do this we need to listen more to what they actually say, rather than speculate about, and then stipulate the significance of, what they might be thought to think.

Interviewees' characterizations of money and markets

Elsewhere I have discussed various aspects of the entanglement of money and eggs in the NESR: whether it is necessarily exploitative, whether it leads to undue inducement, a loss of autonomy and weakened informed consent, and, briefly, whether the entanglement necessarily constitutes the commodification of the human body (Haimes *et al.* 2012; Haimes 2013; Haimes and Taylor 2013). Those papers show that volunteers welcomed the scheme and had no regrets volunteering for it, but were not volunteering under circumstances of their choosing; they would prefer to provide eggs once their own IVF treatment was completed. They volunteered to provide fresh eggs (whose usefulness for their own treatment is therefore unknown at the point of provision) during treatment because of their experiences of the UK IVF bio-economy in which state-funded treatment is difficult to access and private fees are high. The discount was important to their decision to volunteer but not determinative: some withdrew even though that meant they had to pay full fees and almost all declined to donate eggs for the treatment of other couples even though that meant even cheaper fees. The discount was one of a number of complex variables which they juggled in trying to achieve their primary goal of having a baby (Haimes 2013).

In this chapter I focus on how interviewees spoke about the "money and markets" aspects of the scheme. Did they accord the same significance to the issues raised by writers such as Sandel and the Nuffield Council on Bioethics and, if so, how did they navigate their way through them? I first consider how volunteers reasoned through the question of whether they were *selling* their eggs. An American colleague, on hearing about the NESR, commented that "in other words", women were selling their eggs. However, how are such translations into "other words" to be regarded? How are they used, by whom, to make what claims, with what social, legal and moral significance? Did interviewees hear this translation: as a provocation; as a reasonable representation of their actions; as a puzzling characterization; or in some other way? How did they frame and explain their views; what connections did they make or reject; which aspects were they consistent and clear about; what comparisons and contrasts did they draw; which elements did they find challenging, confusing or contradictory? I explore these questions further through an analysis of how interviewees discussed the maximum and minimum amounts of discount they should receive and alternative ways to organize the discounts. To what extent do their views suggest that they regarded themselves as engaging in market-like behaviour?

Are women who participate in the NESR selling their eggs?

I have collected interviewees' views under three broad headings, categorizing ways of discussing this question.

No

Most interviewees were clear, some emphatically, that they were not selling their eggs: "Oh no, definitely not! … [it was] just part of the process … and you just got a little bit of money towards it … I wouldn't just do it to get money" (M09: 663–710).[1] The strength of expression might indicate moral abhorrence but what informs that abhorrence?

One couple introduced the language of "payment" themselves.

THE WOMAN: I didn't actually think of it as "oh well, I'm getting paid for my eggs", I didn't ever feel like that ...

HER PARTNER: I don't think you can put a price on, "here's an egg, there's a £100" ...

THE WOMAN: I don't know {pause} ... I never really thought of it as getting money and selling ... it's like selling a bit of yourself and I've never felt that way. And ... going on the open market, I'd feel a bit like going to the cattle market ...

HER PARTNER: Then it's the highest bidder, isn't it? You may as well put yourself on eBay {laughter}

The direct link between money and eggs invokes associations with "payment" and "selling", yet, importantly, it did not "feel like that" to the couple because they were focused on succeeding with IVF. This exchange displays many of the features apparent in other interviewees' discussions, in distinguishing between what they were doing and what outsiders might regard as selling. For interviewees the idea of selling links to ideas about cash, profit and the initial motivation of "doing it for the money" as opposed to doing it for an entirely different reason.

"I suppose you are selling them, really ..."

Occasionally interviewees edged towards the possibility that the NESR could be defined as selling eggs but embedded that within other factors, including the reasons why they are being sold (if indeed they are), the conditions under which this occurs, and an ongoing interest in what happens to the eggs:

> I don't think egg sharing is selling your eggs, I think it's a way of complementing your fees ... you know where [they're] going to and what's happening with them ... I'm more reassured that whatever's happening in research, you've got some guidelines ... I suppose you are selling them, really, but you're selling them for a better cause.
>
> (M28: 1322–1373)

The implication here is that the NESR simply complements normal IVF. The interviewee sounds defensive and does not explain why she "supposes" it could be selling but if it is to be so defined, it can be justified by the research context.

One woman, acknowledging that she could be seen as selling her eggs because she was engaging in a financial deal, still felt there was a difference: "I suppose it can be seen as selling, you're giving something and you're getting payment for it". She then compared that to selling a DVD on the internet:

> The money I get back for that is not anything specific, it's just cash [but] if I'm giving my eggs for research, the money that's coming back is being used specifically on treatment … You are receiving a payment for doing it, but I can't take that money, put it in my pocket and have a shopping spree … I'm not even getting money back, I'm getting money taken off a bill for treatment and in the same arena. It's the only way I can explain it …
>
> (M27: 1619–1711)

Interviewees felt an implicit criticism in the suggestion that they were selling eggs: "am I selling my eggs? Yeah I probably am and I don't care! {laughter}… But who are these people saying to me 'you're selling your eggs'? Are these people that have never been through this …?" (M05: 1048–1059). Her defensiveness leads her to question the credentials of those raising such issues.

For interviewees, terms such as "selling" do not have simple, uncontested meanings; they reasoned out why the involvement of money might appear to be synonymous with "selling" but, at the same time, why its involvement was experienced differently in these particular circumstances. I shall return to these features in the Commentary, in light of further data. I turn now to consider interviewees' discussions about whether, if the NESR is not defined as selling, they would actually sell their eggs?

Would interviewees sell their eggs?

The extensive distance that most interviewees placed between the NESR and the idea of selling is shown in this discussion. The utterances ranged from brief rejections of the idea – "No, not at all!" (M04: 754–757); "No, never!" (M05: 820–870) – to more detailed considerations. In the latter they deployed a series of distinctions that indicated the boundaries between acceptable and unacceptable transactions around eggs. One said, in reference to selling eggs on the open market,

> No, I don't really agree with that … it's a bit like going abroad and buying a liver isn't it? … I know it's a little bit different but I don't agree … eggs are precious but there [are] ethical things, aren't there … I don't think that's right.

When asked why, she replied,

> I don't know … I feel like it's selling something from my body … I haven't got a big opinion on it because it's just something that I wouldn't do … It's different with research … I feel like I'm doing some good … but

> as for going on the internet and selling your eggs … I don't agree with that … I [would] just feel like I was selling my body.
>
> (M02: 704–748)

Interviewees used the internet as short-hand for the open market. One illustrated the stylistic tropes that others used when she joked: "I wouldn't put them on eBay! No. But a proper clinic …" (M26: 818–839). She later emphasized, "No, not the internet, no. Maybe if times get hard! {laughing}" (M26: 1175–1182). The use of joking suggests unease with both the idea of selling and with the involvement of the internet. Another compared selling eggs on the internet to selling to "back street butchers", conflating the two charges normally levelled at illegal abortionists, of operating in dubious unhygienic settings and using poor quality, physically damaging, techniques, suggesting her strength of feeling about this possibility (M27: 1523–1585).

Concerns were raised about what would happen to the eggs if they were sold over the internet:

> My fear would be "what are they going to be used for?" whereas I felt confident that my eggs were going to be used with the [clinic] as they said they were going to be used … it goes back to trusting what's going to happen to them … {sigh, pause}… it doesn't seem {pause} as comfortable as sharing your eggs through a process that you're already doing.
>
> (M11: 921–941)

"A process that you're already doing", similar to the earlier phrase, "in the same arena", implies associating with places, people and purposes already known and accepted, whereas the internet is associated with the unknown.

One woman expressed the views raised by others when asked what she thought of a system where women were given £1,500 cash for eggs and could decide for themselves how they wanted to use it:

> to me that puts it in the same category of stories you hear about people in America or in third world countries where they sell their … organs … where do you draw the line? What if you have a drug addict who's desperate for money and so they'll donate you 50% of their eggs … [what] if it was an alcoholic ?

It is right to target IVF patients, "because it's women who are in this who understand why you need [eggs] and I think anybody else would only do it for the money and I think that's when it becomes unethical" (M25: 972–1025). IVF patients provide eggs, "for all the right reasons" (M27: 1619–1741). That the use of cash might produce certain consequences, including attracting the wrong sort of donors, encapsulates interviewees' views on why the NESR is not seen as selling and what could happen if it were to be "more like" selling.

Should egg providers receive a "fee per egg" instead?

I asked interviewees whether the reduced fees discount could be packaged in any other way, to see what priorities, limits and boundaries were expressed. For example, would they prefer a system in which they were given a fee for each egg, rather than a fixed discount, regardless of the number of eggs provided? As can be seen above, the idea of deciding a specified sum of money for a single egg was taken as partly definitive of "selling" but was also something that was often raised as presenting a conceptual, moral and practical obstacle to actually selling. Perhaps not surprisingly then, most interviewees rejected the suggestion of a fee per egg. However, the grounds they gave for doing so proved very interesting given that their reasons for participating in the NESR in the first place were to access cheaper IVF cycles.

Interviewees forcibly rejected the "fee per egg" suggestion because it was unfair, as the number of eggs a woman produced was not under her control and no one could do anything extra to produce more and "earn" a bigger discount. As one said, deploying a phrase that shows how difficult IVF treatment is, "[they are all] going through the same trauma however many eggs they are producing" (M18: 748–780). Similarly, others said, "you can't do anything more than what your body will let you do" (M26: 1107–1173) and "it's not up to you, you can't do anything about it. No, it should be the same. Price per egg is wrong {laughing}" (M22: 939–954).

Interviewees also argued that a "fee per egg" system would put IVF patients under additional pressure, especially if it meant that they could only afford another IVF cycle by producing a certain number of eggs:

> you're under so much pressure to produce as many eggs as you can [in IVF] … I wouldn't like the pressure then of saying each egg was worth £250 or something [compared with] the guarantee that you were going to get £1,500 to be able to afford the cycle … 'Cos if you didn't get that many eggs, how are you going to pay for the rest of the cycle?
>
> (M11: 954–985).

Interestingly, one woman, when asked about "fee per egg", immediately clarified, "You buy each egg?", then reasoned,

> Erm, {long pause}, no I don't think that's fair … if someone who isn't lucky enough to produce so many eggs, gets less money or less of a chance [of pregnancy] than someone who does produce a lot of eggs, just 'cos they're unfortunate enough to not have so many eggs, it doesn't make their sacrifice any less, well it's harder for them really to make that decision than someone who produces a lot of eggs.
>
> (M07: 712–747)

This use of "sacrifice" echoes comments elsewhere in the interviews that women would prefer to give eggs after they had achieved a pregnancy rather than during their IVF treatment.

For interviewees, as IVF patients, the value of eggs is calculated in relation to the eggs' contributions to increasing the chances of pregnancy. In general, interviewees thought that more eggs could mean more chances of pregnancy but they also knew that an exceptionally high number of eggs does not have a proportionately increased effect on those chances, so if one has 40 eggs, giving away 20 is unlikely to reduce those chances significantly whereas giving away two out of four eggs is much more likely to do so. Eggs, in and of themselves, are not regarded as having any innate value or price; rather, eggs have a dual worth, representing both the chances of pregnancy and the chances of more treatment; both are important to interviewees. From this perspective, the involvement of money neither erodes nor increases the "preciousness" of eggs; similarly, exchanging eggs for more treatment does not devalue those eggs (Haimes 2013). The "fee per egg" suggestion was not objected to on the moral grounds that this would be more like selling, or "purchase", as defined by the Nuffield Council on Bioethics (2011) but on two different and associated grounds: that of the practical goals of reducing stress during IVF, and that of fairness, within the arduous IVF process of producing those eggs.

Interviewees' responses to the "fee per egg" suggestion display several features: first, the fact that none of them had suggested such a scheme themselves indicates that they were not motivated by the wish to maximize their income from their eggs; second, it elicited references to their not being in control of the processes of producing eggs; third, that lack of control meant that it was not in their power to produce more eggs; and, fourth, that then elicited highly moral discourses around "fairness", "earning", "deserving". The language of fairness could be partly defensive as interviewees do not know how many eggs they will produce in any particular cycle and they would not want to be someone who gets less of a discount. Nonetheless, this is such a recurrent, and strongly emphatic, feature of their talk that there is clearly a pervasive concern for others like themselves who are going through IVF.

Maximum and minimum amounts for the discount

I asked interviewees about their sense of acceptable and unacceptable maximum and minimum levels of discount on IVF treatment for providing eggs to research. This helped to tease out whether they had strong views about the actual figures offered or about what their eggs are "worth" and whether they volunteered for the NESR wanting to negotiate good terms for themselves. Interviewees generally liked the rough, though inaccurate (because total IVF fees have increased whereas the discount has remained at £1,500) symmetry of 50 per cent eggs for 50 per cent discount. One interviewee, when asked: "So they took half your eggs?" replied, "Yeah and I paid half the money and I think that's quite fair" (M22: 925–941).

Although interviewees were uncomfortable discussing specific sums of money – "it sounds awful … it's not all about the money" (M02: 779–806) – a clear sense of what would be too low emerged, judged in relation to the full IVF price and their chances of more treatment. When asked if £500 would have been enough, one replied, "probably not, no {laughing} … But half price for us was great, we can get another round of treatment in" (M05: 909–940). Another picked out her own figure for what would be too low: "it's not very nice having your eggs retrieved. I think £1,500 is quite a reasonable amount … I wouldn't do it for £50! Oh my God, no! {laughs}" (M26: 870–891). Commonly £500 was a figure mentioned as not being enough, either because that was a sum they could imagine raising from elsewhere without having to contemplate giving up some of their eggs or because that would buy an insufficient portion of an additional cycle of treatment. Interviewees also identified dangers in offering too high a discount.

> I think any more than [£1,500] and you might end up with any Tom, Dick or Harry coming through the door … you end up with the wrong type of people coming in for treatment … people who are only in it for the money and are only in it for the reduced cost.
>
> (M04: 762–806)

In brief, interviewees valued the discount for its ability to increase their chances of private IVF treatment, not as a sum of money in its own right; as with the discussion on selling, they were keen to establish that they were not volunteering for the NESR "for the money" but within a context in which they could gain something for themselves and give something back. Embarrassment when discussing money in detail might be partly because in the UK we are not used to discussing money in relation to health care; these comments might be "heard" differently elsewhere. Nonetheless this is evidence that money was troubling and that interviewees were keen to establish certain views about the different types of money being made available and discussed.

Commentary

There are several claims in the interviews about what the NESR is, and what it is not, in the ways in which money features in its transactions. In supposing, sometimes reluctantly, that the NESR "must" amount to the selling of eggs simply because it is (amongst other things) a financial transaction, interviewees are reflecting Strathern's (2012) observation that in many debates, when money enters the room, all other considerations fly out of the window. However, in also resisting that easy and singular association between money and selling, and by focusing on those "other things that it is amongst", interviewees are also demonstrating that everyday life, and the role of money within it, is somewhat more nuanced and complex than usually supposed (Zelizer 1997; Almeling 2011).

It is not easy to resist that singular association, as can be seen by the style in which interviewees seek to articulate their views. They pause, hesitate and joke as they stress how their experiences *feel* different to other apparently more authoritative claims and they seek ways of mitigating what they hear as criticism, or even accusation, of selling. Jokes expressed the outer limits of what might be deemed acceptable: one cannot possibly auction eggs on eBay. The interviewees, while actively seeking a discount on their IVF fees, are nonetheless troubled by money.

Zelizer (1997, 2) observes that money is commonly thought to create cold personal relationships and not surprisingly (since interviewees encounter those views in all sorts of aspects of their lives) some of those fears are heard in the quotations above. It is partly because of this standard view that Sandel (2012), as one of its proponents, can blur his use of terms such as "money", "markets", "buying" and "selling" as if these have commonly accepted and almost interchangeable meanings. However, Zelizer's riposte is that people introduce all sorts of distinctions about how money operates in their everyday lives: "distinction and multiplication appear on every hand" (Zelizer 1997, 4). This reflects more closely interviewees' reasoning on these issues: we can identify a range of distinctions that they draw and can show how those link to, and bump up against, other ideas, to see which distinctions matter, and in what ways. At least five lines of distinction emerge in interviewees' discourses on ideas around eggs, money and selling.

The IVF context

We have argued elsewhere (Haimes *et al.* 2012) that the IVF context is highly influential on the interviewees' framing of their experiences: they are only involved in the NESR because they are IVF patients and because their overriding goal is to have a baby. This framing encompasses their orientations towards the role of money in those experiences, including their views that there should be more state funding of IVF and that private fees are too high (Haimes 2013). It is not surprising then that the IVF context shapes some of their views on whether the NESR constitutes egg selling. A key distinction that they draw, in asserting a difference between the NESR and selling, is that, in participating in the NESR, they are not doing anything much different from "normal IVF"; it is "part of the process", "in the same arena" as their treatment. The meaning and value of eggs are calculated with reference to the chances of success in their own IVF treatment, in which the open market is deemed irrelevant. Participation in the NESR is not "about" the money but "about" getting treatment and having a baby and they would not be providing their eggs other than to get cheaper treatment. It does not feel like selling because their subjective motivation lies in a completely different direction and social domain.

The importance of the IVF context in framing their views of the relationship between money and eggs is most clearly seen in interviewees' comments on the "fee per egg" suggestion. Their concerns switch from distancing themselves from the idea of selling to aligning themselves with other women also undergoing IVF, where every egg counts. The potential unfairness of "fee per egg", plus its likely impact in increasing stress, anxiety and poor responses to treatment, completely negates other considerations and it was firmly rejected. Although Weber describes money as "impersonal" and Simmel asserts its "heartlessness" (Zelizer 1997, 6) neither resonates with interviewees' discussions about a "fee per egg"; rather, they display a concern for others and for fairness rather than for maximizing their own gains over others. Such a unanimous, other-concerned, response counters Sandel's pessimism about money driving out altruistic concerns; the data considered here suggest that whether or not this happens depends on how the money is embedded, and acted upon, within specific socio-cultural contexts. The interviews support the Nuffield Council on Bioethics' (2011) assertion of the importance of context, and fill in the details lacking in that report, by providing indications of the discursive practices through which relevant contexts are constituted and deployed as both a topic and a resource for reasoning.

The nature of the money that is or is not involved

One of the characteristics of debates about money is the assumption that "money" is a single, uncontested, entity, but we have already seen Zelizer's (1997, 2) suggestion that in everyday life all sorts of distinctions are drawn between types of money. This is clearly the case for these interviewees. While some move towards saying that the NESR is egg selling because it is a financial transaction, they and others also suggest that the money involved in the NESR has distinctive features that differentiate it from the money involved in selling. For example, the NESR money is not "cash" or a "profit" or a "cheque" or "disposable income" or "earnings" or "money back"; it is "money off" and it is "half price". Also it is money directed towards a specific use, as a "means to an end", for accessing further, cheaper, treatment; the money, as Zelizer (1997) would say, is "earmarked" and not transferable to other activities, such as a shopping spree. These distinctions establish that whilst some transactions involving money might be problematic, the particular transaction around the NESR is morally acceptable.

The references by some interviewees to how money in the form of cash might attract the wrong people for the wrong reasons reflects Almeling's (2011) argument that we should look at how, and what type of, money actually changes hands in the gamete market, to understand how the transaction is experienced and understood by those involved (clinicians as well as gamete providers). As our analysis shows, attention to contextual detail is important; it might be partly because actual money does not change hands in the NESR that interviewees are able to make some of these distinctions.

Interviewees' discursive practices reflect the Nuffield Council on Bioethics' (2011, 4) contention that "money may be conceptualised in many ways" though they do not echo the neatness of the report's monetary typology. The report is written broadly from the perspectives of state agencies and research bodies concerned to find ethical means of promoting the safe contribution of human materials to treatment and research; one can only speculate how its register, and categorical distinctions, might differ if written from the perspective of actual and potential providers of those bodily materials.

Not participating in market-like behaviour

Interviewees did not see themselves as engaging in market-like behaviours. Beyond the practical difficulty of not knowing how to participate in the market, even if they had wanted to, they argued, implicitly and explicitly, that their actions and motivations distinguished them from those operating in the market place. For example, going into the market presumes a profit motivation, "doing it for the money", which all denied; rather, they were participating in the NESR mostly to help themselves and partly to help research. Orienting their actions towards an unseen, third-party beneficiary ("research") rather than towards personal profit was how many interviewees expressed their lack of interest in the open market.

Market behaviour also requires detailed calculations of a price for the goods in terms of what the market will bear, but no interviewee could see how to put a price on an egg, let alone proposed a rationale for one price over another. The "fee per egg" suggestion would have been an opportunity to do this but instead interviewees directed the discussion towards the unfairness of such proposals. Similarly, the discussion around maximum and minimum levels of discounts produced very few examples of specific sums of money, particularly at the higher end. Interviewees' assertions that they were not seeking a profit or a surplus are supported by the nature of their discussion in these areas. Also, as several said, laughing about going on eBay, they were not interested in selling their eggs to the highest bidder, a practice that would be definitive of market-like behaviour. Similarly, the fact that eggs cannot be appropriately compared with DVDs underscores the absence of any market-like behaviour amongst interviewees, since the market depends on a notion of the lack of difference between goods and their essential sameness as commodities. Also none bargained for an actual 50 per cent fees discount even though they struggled to pay private IVF fees and with the "monied" world of IVF in general.

This appears to be how interviewees address Sandel's (2012, 79) challenge of how to decide whether to participate in "morally questionable markets"; interviewees clearly do link market reasoning with moral reasoning. However, their distancing of themselves from market-like behaviour is in many ways curious because it is in marked contrast to the ways in which the market place for IVF treatment, in which they find themselves, operates (Winston 2011). Nonetheless, as reflexive actors, interviewees are constituting both the contexts of relevance for their actions while at the same time constituting themselves as certain types of persons; in this case, persons who do not see themselves as traders in the market place for human eggs.

The "location" of the transaction

Interviewees' perceptions of the degrading nature of the market are seen in the comparisons they draw with places like cattle markets: cold, dirty, noisy, lacking human dignity and focused on auctioneering for the highest price. Similarly, the reference made to places like "backstreet butchers" conveys the strength of concern about just where, and how, any market in eggs would function. References to the internet elicited further concerns about a lack of regulation and whether using the internet would be an explicit venture into the open market. The internet's market goals, practices and consequences, were contrasted with the NESR's goals, practices and consequences.

A key factor for interviewees in distinguishing participation in the NESR from participation in the open market is that the NESR transaction takes place in "the clinic", either the clinic they know from previous treatments or the clinic they "know" as an abstract but nonetheless "proper" place. This is contrasted with the internet, and occasionally "abroad", "America", the "third world", which are all seen as odd, "out of place", alien locations, unregulated and managed by unknown people, as far as any dealings around eggs are concerned and which thereby transform any transaction accordingly. The synecdochal reference to the "clinic" indicates all that is right about the experience: it is clean, familiar, regulated, staffed with "proper" doctors and nurses who know what they are doing and who can be trusted, and attended by women who have a better understanding than others of just what eggs mean. The clinic also has "proper" reasons for encouraging this transaction, assisting the "good cause" of research. Interviewees' utterances convey the idea of the clinic as a socially, physically and, most important, *morally* comfortable place in which transactions around eggs should occur.

The concern with the "location" of the transaction suggests that the introduction of money via the NESR is made possible and acceptable through *existing* social relationships: partly through pre-existing associations between IVF and money, but mostly through pre-existing interpersonal relationships between the patient and clinic staff, plus the location of the clinic within the familiar institution of the National Health Service. As far as the NESR is concerned, social relationships are not being eroded by money, as is often assumed, but are the very element that makes the involvement of money possible in the first place. As Zelizer (1997, 18–21) observes, it is not the case that money necessarily flattens or corrodes social relationships, as is assumed in classic Marxist analyses, but this can only be understood if we explore how markets are actually organized and experienced (Almeling 2011).

Retaining an interest in their eggs

Zelizer (1997, 7–8) also challenges Marxist assumptions that money alienates subjective connections between individuals and the objects they produce and reduces all personal relations to the "*cash nexus*". Interviewees' discursive practices support Zelizer's challenge: part of their concern about selling eggs on the open market is that they would not know what happened to them and they fear that they could be misused. It is not the case that once they receive the discount they no longer care about their eggs. As we have seen, it also matters that the scheme is provided by an organization that they know. This illustrates further that, far from being obliterated by the offer of a discount, subjective connections are *central* to the process of volunteering for the NESR.

Interviewees perceive their eggs as not easily separable from themselves and their bodies. While eggs might be physically separable (IVF relies on that) they are not morally separable; interviewees retain a sense of responsibility towards their eggs, even after donation. They emphasized the similarity between their eggs and other body parts and talked of eggs as being part of their bodies and indeed part of their selves. They did not distinguish between the characteristics of eggs and other body parts along the commonly accepted lines of: multiple eggs/single organs; reproductive tissue/non-reproductive tissue; use for treatment/research. Rather, in discussions around money, they emphasized how the eggs relate to, and are understood with reference to, the whole body. This is an apparent contradiction to the suggestion elsewhere (Haimes 2013) that the IVF process emphasizes the entification of eggs and their exchangeability. However, what appears to be the case for interviewees is that eggs can be detached and exchanged to achieve the goal of having a baby but not for lesser goals like making money. In other words, there is entification of eggs in IVF, but this is not necessarily true of all eggs in all situations; only in certain contexts do eggs become entities, at other times they are not only part of the body but also part of the self. Thus, whilst Sandel (2012) is concerned that the very fact of exchange taints that which is being exchanged, the interviewees demonstrate that, in the case of eggs at least, "that which is being exchanged" does not have one single, stable definition, let alone one single, stable status, financial or moral.

To return to the original concerns that provoked these discussions: does the entanglement of money and eggs constitute the commodification of bodily parts, and therefore the marketization of such transactions, and is this a "bad thing"? One can understand the genuine socio-moral concerns that lead writers such as Sandel (2012) to answer "yes" to all three questions (Strathern 2012). However, interviewees' accounts suggest that more complex understandings of the many varied relationships between money and body parts are possible and necessary; the meanings and actions attached to, and around, "money" are not straightforward. The relationship is neither linear nor causal and the debates therefore cannot easily settle into either "pro" or "anti" the involvement of money in such transactions. Instead we need to follow Hoeyer's (2013, 3) suggestion to think "about value in a way that combines moral and epistemological dimensions with the notion of monetary worth, but we must do so reflectively and without presuming too much about what money does and what bodies are". The interviews reported on in this chapter reinforce the need to examine *particular* cases of entanglement closely, as well as the need to interrogate key terms, such as markets, commodification and most of all, "money", even more closely.

Thanks

With thanks to the interviewees, Erik Malmqvist, Kristin Zeiler, Robin Williams, Ken Taylor, Alison Murdoch, the Newcastle Fertility Centre and the Medical Research Council (grant G0701109).

Note

1 The M number is the unique identifier allocated to each interviewee. It is followed by line numbers that indicate the location of the quoted passage in the interview transcript.

References

Almeling, R. 2011. *Sex Cells: The Medical Market for Eggs and Sperm*. Berkeley: University of California Press.

Braun, K., and S. Schulz. 2012. "Oocytes for Research." *New Genetics and Society* 32: 135–157.

Egli, D., Chen, A., Saphier, G., Powers, D., Alper, M., and K. Katz. 2011. "Impracticality of Egg Donor Recruitment in the Absence of Compensation." *Cell Stem Cell* 9: 293–294.

Haimes, E. 2013. "Juggling on a Rollercoaster? Gains, Loss and Uncertainties in IVF Patients' Accounts of Volunteering for a U.K. 'Egg Sharing for Research' Scheme." *Social Science and Medicine* 86: 45–51.

Haimes, E., and K. Taylor. 2013. "What Is the Role of Reduced IVF Fees in Persuading Women to Volunteer to Provide Eggs for Research?" *Human Fertility* 16: 246–251.

Haimes, E., Taylor, K., and I. Turkmendag. 2012. "Eggs, Ethics and Exploitation?" *Sociology of Health and Illness* 34: 1199–1214.

Haimes, E., Skene, L., Ballantyne, A., Caulfield, T., Goldstein, L., Hyun, I., Kimmelman, J., Robert, J., Scott, C., Solbakk, J.H., Sugarman, J., Taylor, P., and G. Testa. 2013. "ISSCR Ethics and Public Policy Committee: Position Statement on the Provision and Procurement of Human Eggs for Stem Cell Research." *Cell Stem Cell* 12: 285–291.

Hamm, D., and J. Anton. 2012. "Donor Compensation." *Human Reproduction* 27(suppl 2): ii32–;ii34.

HFEA (Human Fertilisation and Embryology Authority). 2006. *Donating Eggs for Research*. London: HFEA.

Hoeyer, K. 2013. *Exchanging Human Bodily Material*. Dordrecht: Springer.

Noggle, S., Fung, H.-L., Gore, A., Martinez, H., Satriani, K.C., Prosser, R., Oum, K., Paull, D., Druckenmiller, S., and M. Freeby. 2011. "Human Oocytes Reprogram Somatic Cells to a Pluripotent State." *Nature* 478: 70–75.

Nuffield Council on Bioethics. 2011. *Human Bodies: Donation for Medicine and Research*. London: Nuffield Council on Bioethics.

Pattinson, S. 2012. "The Value of Bodily Material." *Medical Law Review* 20: 576–603.

Radin, M.J. 1996. *Contested Commodities.* Cambridge: Harvard University Press.

Roberts, C., and K. Throsby. 2008. "Paid to Share." *Social Science & Medicine* 66: 159–169.

Roxland, B. 2012. "New York State's Landmark Policies on Oversight and Compensation for Egg Donation to Stem Cell Research." *Regenerative Medicine* 7: 397–408.

Sandel, M. 2012. *What Money Can't Buy.* London: Allen Lane.

Strathern, M. 2012. "Gifts Money Cannot Buy." *Social Anthropology* 20: 397–410.

Svenaeus, F. 2010. "The Body as Gift, Resource or Commodity?" *Journal of Bioethical Inquiry* 7: 163–172.

Waldby, C., and K. Carroll. 2012. "Egg Donation for Stem Cell Research." *Sociology of Health and Illness* 34: 513–528.

Waldby, C., Kerridge, I., Boulos, M., and K. Carroll. 2013. "From Altruism to Monetisation." *Social Science & Medicine* 94: 34–42.

Winston, R. 2011. "Public Bodies Bill: Third Reading, House of Lords." *Hansard,* May 9th, col: 693.

Zelizer, V.A. 1997. *The Social Meaning of Money.* Princeton: Princeton University Press.

5 Sharing organs for transplantation

Altruism as *kagandahang loob*

Leonardo D. de Castro

Introduction

This chapter seeks to understand "sharing" in the context of organ transplantation by exploring how it can be contrasted with the generic concept of "giving". The starting point is an analysis of ethical concepts within the framework of Filipino culture as this informs the understanding of meanings and expectations associated with the concept of *utang na loob* (debt of good will).

By making a comparison with material debt such as that which is incurred when a bank loan is taken out the chapter seeks to further clarify essential features of *utang na loob* that are not ordinarily associated with purely material indebtedness. Then it examines concomitant relationships and expectations as well as the implications that these have for the understanding of organ donation. In the end, the chapter shows that prevailing paradigms of altruism that currently determine what is ethically acceptable are too rigid and narrow in that they fail to accommodate well-meaning offers of organ donation.

Giving and the significance of roles

There are many types of situations when someone can be said to give something. Various acts of giving can be differentiated by these types and by the roles that givers and recipients assume. The significance of particular acts of giving can best be understood when these differences are sorted out. The same needs to be said about understanding the significance of particular cases of organ donation. Furthermore, different people have different roles to play in various giving contexts.

Organ donation for transplantation is a kind of giving that does not easily fit into a single paradigm. Disagreements regarding ethically appropriate ways of soliciting or donating organs for transplant have led some people to believe that there must be a single correct paradigm that is applicable – based on altruism – and that givings that do not fit that paradigm are suspect. People in different circumstances do not always agree on what altruism should be taken to mean but the view appears to be prevalent that altruistic donation requires the absence of payment or monetary consideration (Participants in the International Summit on Transplant Tourism and Organ Trafficking 2008; WHO 2010; WMA 2014).

The discussion of acts of good will and debts of good will shows that altruism need not always be defined in terms of the absence of payment or the expectation thereof. Altruistic giving takes place in different socio-cultural contexts and one must understand a specific context as well as the roles played by people in that context in order to appreciate the significance of a specific act of giving. By understanding the roles that people play in such situations one begins to appreciate that an act of giving is, more importantly, an act of sharing. Sharing takes place within a socio-cultural context that defines the nature of roles and relationships. This chapter explores a particular context that revolves around the Filipino concept of *kagandahang loob* (roughly, good will) and *utang na loob* (Kaut 1961; Hollnsteiner 1973; Befu 1977, 259; de Castro 1998).

Debts of gratitude, debts of good will

Debts of gratitude are those that are incurred by people who receive help or favours from others in times of acute need. The indebtedness is understood to extend beyond the material equivalent of actual benefits received. In recognizing a debt of gratitude, one also recognizes the good will manifested by the benefactor in providing assistance or granting a favour. For this reason, this chapter refers to *utang na loob* as "debt of good will" instead of as "debt of gratitude". The former terminology focuses attention on a critical feature of the concept that "debt of gratitude" fails to capture. That critical feature is the *kagandahang loob* (good will) that accompanies the external assistance or favour given.

A closer look at monetary debt enables us to show how a debt of good will is different and how its features give rise to certain expectations within the context of social relationships. We are also able eventually to examine the implications of these relationships and expectations for the understanding of organ donation.

Monetary debt

When a person owes money to a bank, it is usually the result of an act of borrowing. The transaction would be an institutional one in the sense of being governed by policies and regulations defined by the lending institution. Prospective borrowers are informed of the specific terms of indebtedness. In the end, the borrower is expected to know the exact amount that needs to be paid back in order for the indebtedness to be cleared. When the complete amount is paid back no indebtedness remains.

Indebtedness of good will is not framed within a context of regulations defined by an institution. When a debt of good will is incurred, there is no entity that corresponds to a bank in a money lending transaction.

Nevertheless, there is an indebtedness that is created and is waiting to be repaid. Rather than formal regulations, there are socio-cultural values that define expectations and help us to understand the nature of debts of good will and the circumstances under which people incur such debts or are expected to repay them.

Organ donation as a debt of good will

When someone receives a kidney donation for transplantation, a debt of good will is incurred. It is an event that creates expectations for "repayment". By itself, the receipt of assistance or favour does not put the recipient in a position of indebtedness of good will. Debts of good will are incurred when the beneficiary is in acute need of the assistance given or favour granted. The debt could then be appreciated as one of good will because, by catering to another person's pressing need, the benefactor is able to help fulfil that need and convey *kagandahang loob* (good will) towards the beneficiary.

What happens then is not only a giving of help. The act of helping serves as a vehicle for empathy or concern. The benefactor is not only giving something that is external to him. In a manner of speaking, he is also able to give of himself. It is in this regard that the organ donor not only gives, but also shares.

Sharing of oneself: creating a debt of good will

When a bank loan has been repaid, the borrower has complied with his obligations. It would not make sense to talk about a debt of good will. The situation would be different when a person borrows money from a neighbour who usually is not engaged in the business of lending money. The neighbour is giving more than the amount of money that he is making available to the borrower. He is sharing part of himself.

The Filipino term *utang na loob* literally means indebtedness of one's *kalooban* (inner self). In the case of an organ donation, the donor conveys *kagandahang loob* and shares of herself. Because the donor shares good will, good will is what she is owed. It is the act of sharing of oneself that creates an *utang na loob*. The act of sharing needs to be repaid, usually through another act of sharing. In material terms, there is no formula to determine the amount that needs to be repaid as "quantification is undefined" (Panopio and Rolda 2006, 86). There are no time limits for settling the obligation. There are no explicit rules to determine these parameters.

There is another feature that it is important to understand in this connection – in the socio-cultural context in which indebtedness of will thrives, it is not recognized as correct for the person who has given a favour to demand that she be materially reciprocated. A person who demands material reciprocation is *materyoso*, which is a negative word to describe someone who unacceptably focuses on the material or external value of her contribution rather than on the internal *kagandahang loob*. Making such a demand also establishes the person's preoccupation with repayment and the lack of *kusang loob* (free will) because of the material motivation. After all, the key component of the favour is good will rather than something of material value. In the case of an organ donation for transplant, it is the benefactor's *kagandahang loob* that creates the *utang na loob*.

Interestingly, while it is not for the original benefactor to demand reciprocation – because acts of good will are not done with the expectation of reward – there is nevertheless another source of expectation that the beneficiary should be willing to repay in some way. This source is the social community that regards commitment to repay as a virtue. The recipient of good will must be ready to give of herself in return when the opportunity arises. It is not a matter of personal obligation to the benefactor.

The expectation to repay is not something that arises in the context of a one-time reciprocal relationship between the benefactor and the beneficiary. Rather, it arises as a societal expectation. The willingness and readiness to repay indebtedness of good will is a virtue – it is a trait that has come to be regarded as essential for human flourishing within that society. This does not mean that the material benefit is unimportant or that it can totally be ignored. In the context of debts of good will, the material benefit takes on an extra-material dimension provided by the sharing context.

Confirming a relationship between benefactor and beneficiary

To speak of indebtedness of will on the part of an organ recipient is to take into account the prior existence or establishment of a socio-cultural relationship within which repayment can take place and be understood. We examine further the nature of this relationship by trying to understand what it means for someone to be *walang utang na loob* (roughly, ingrate).

One of the worst things that can be said of a Filipino as an ethical commentary is that he is *walang utang na loob* – that is to say, he fails to recognize indebtedness of will. He fails to see himself as being situated in a relationship of *pakikipagkapwa* (roughly, solidarity) that comes with his indebtedness of will. In the case of a beneficiary of an organ donation, he fails to recognize how important it is for him to have been the beneficiary of the donation and how significant the donor's good will has been in improving his condition. Beyond describing what he does or fails to do, to say that someone is *walang utang na loob* is to make an ethical judgment of the person – it is to say that he has an unsavoury character, that he is acting shamefully, or worse, that he could even be failing to recognize his shameful behaviour.

In contrast, one who recognizes indebtedness of will is expected to be mindful of the needs of a person that he is indebted to. Hence, the recipient of an organ donated for transplantation is expected to look after the urgent needs of her benefactor. This is neither something that needs to be demanded of him as a matter of compensation nor something that is merely a matter of contractual reciprocity. Rather, this is a matter of recognizing a need for a virtuous response to good will manifested by the organ donor. Being more than a case of giving, the sharing of oneself requires a reciprocal sharing of oneself with the other who is regarded as similar and equal.

Debt of good will and *hiya* (moral shame)

Closely related to the concept of a debt of good will is the Filipino sense of *hiya* (roughly, moral shame). It is important to understand three points about *hiya*:

1 Regardless of the specific meaning of *hiya* in a particular context, it has a relational character. Shame and humiliation could be felt in relation to one person or to the public in general.
2 In ordinary language use, *nakakahiya* (roughly, shameful) is more commonly used than the Filipino equivalents of "bad", "wrong", or "evil" to express moral or ethical disapproval. One would more often say "Don't do that – that is shameful!" than "Don't do that – that is bad!". And even when someone says, "That is bad!" one would not be surprised to observe that this expression is used almost interchangeably with "That is shameful!" or "You ought to be ashamed of yourself for doing that!".
3 *Hiya* is intimately related to indebtedness of will.

The first two points highlight the relational character of *hiya* and the central place that *hiya* has in Filipino ethical ontology. The third point requires greater elaboration. For example:

> Failure to discharge the payment [for *utang na loob*] causes *hiya*, and one who does not recognize *utang na loob* is considered as *walang hiya* (showing no shame) … When an individual cannot reciprocate the favor done to him, … *hiya* is the usual reaction … there is the *walang hiya* kind of person who does not fulfill his obligation of *utang na loob.*
>
> (Panopio and Rolda 2006, 86)

Hiya relates to indebtedness of will in that indebtedness of will entails an obligation on the part of the "debtor" that is founded on *hiya*. A debtor, i.e. a recipient of an urgent favour from a benefactor, is bound by a relationship of *hiya* to society, to repay the favour received from the benefactor. To be *walang utang na loob*, then, is to be *walang hiya*, i.e. to be morally deficient. To call a Filipino *walang hiya*, or "shameless", "is to wound him seriously … " (Hollnsteiner 1973, 75).

While the specific origin of indebtedness is the benefactor, the obligation to repay is an obligation to society more broadly. The *hiya* arises as a response to social norms but is more than the mere feeling of shame that one may experience. It has been defined as "the uncomfortable feeling that accompanies awareness of being in a socially unacceptable position, or performing a socially unacceptable action" (Lynch 1962, 97). It has also been described as "like fear or a sense of inadequacy and anxiety in an uncontrolled and threatening situation" (Bulatao 1964, 426). It includes a sensitivity to the possibility of moral rebuke.

At a minimum, an *utang na loob* has to be recognized and acknowledged, if not repaid. This minimum can be acceptable because, understandably, not all of those who owe debts of good will are in a position to repay – at least not immediately or not in a timely or adequate way. But the recognition and acknowledgement of that indebtedness have to be present: "The acceptance of the *kabubut-on* [*kagandahang loob* in Cebuano language] (gift of oneself) … implies that the receiver is willing and eager to help the giver when the latter's need for help arises" (Quisumbing 1976, 262).

Organ sharing as altruism

The sharing of oneself in organ donation can be seen as an act of altruism within the given socio-cultural milieu. What this means can be better appreciated if one understands the conditions under which an agent can be said to act out of good will.

An act can be considered to convey *kagandahang loob* only if it is done (1) out of *kusang loob* (roughly, voluntarily) and thus, not under external compulsion, (2) while being motivated by positive feelings (e.g. charity, love or empathy) for the beneficiary, and (3) without being motivated by the anticipation of reward.

It is important for the agent to be acting without external compulsion because the desire to benefit others must arise as an unsolicited autonomous initiative. The good will must flow spontaneously and without the agent having to be told to do what needs to be done. Willingness to comply with the expectations of others would not suffice. It is important for *kagandahang loob* that beneficial acts be initiated by the agent without having to be solicited by others. An agent must also be motivated by genuine feelings for the beneficiaries of his actions. There can be no *kagandahang loob* if a person performs his duties without positive emotional involvement.

Actions done in anticipation of reward or personal gain are not done out of *kusang loob.* There can be no *kagandahang loob* if actions are tainted by a selfish desire. If one's beneficial actions are calculated to gain public recognition or material reward, they lose the purity that is essential to *kagandahang loob.*

The three conditions identified constitute necessary requirements for *kagandahang loob.* Some would say that if providing assistance could not be done without meeting these requirements, it would be better for the assistance not to be given at all, no matter how beneficial it might be. The intended recipient may refuse the offering of assistance if that assistance is not being given out of *kusang loob.* In this sense, the conveyance of *kagandahang loob* is more valuable than the benefits arising from a supposedly "altruistic" act.

If an organ donation were to be seen as an altruistic act within this context, it has to satisfy the three conditions mentioned above. The organ donor must (1) not be acting under external compulsion, (2) be motivated by positive feelings (e.g. charity, love or empathy) toward the beneficiary, and (3) not be motivated by an expectation of reward. These same three conditions are the reasons why an altruistic organ donation constitutes not only an act of giving but of sharing. The donation involves not only the handing over of something material but the conveyance of *kagandahang loob* under circumstances that establish an ethics-based relationship characterized by solidarity involving the beneficiary and benefactor.

Implications for compensation and incentives

Given the above characterization of *kagandahang loob*, it seems that compensation and incentives would have no place in the understanding of altruistic organ donation. Taking these material considerations into account means that an agent acts under external compulsion. Although the donor could still be motivated by positive feelings toward the beneficiary, it is difficult to see how the third condition (the lack of anticipation of reward or personal gain) could still be satisfied. Moreover, if the prospective donor acts out of *kusang loob*, she could not expect, much less demand, reciprocal treatment by the beneficiary. *Kagandahang loob* presupposes disinterest in compensation or reward for the beneficial act.

Nevertheless, there are three factors that complicate the situation and give rise to the conclusion that the recipient still has the obligation to repay the debt. First, there is something that needs to be repaid – the *kagandahang loob*. Second, there is a sense of moral shame that relates to an expectation by society that the beneficiary will repay when the opportunity arises. This second factor further leads to a third, which involves the beneficiary's character – the virtue that lies in the ability to recognize indebtedness of will. In this kind of context then, there arises a situation where, on the one hand, the organ donor does not have a right to expect reciprocation but, on the other hand, the organ recipient has an obligation to repay the indebtedness of will. Because of the three factors mentioned above, classification into altruistic or non-altruistic does not necessarily serve to establish whether an organ donation should be acceptable or not. For example, organ donors may be given post-donation rewards that come to them as a complete surprise. They may be purely and properly motivated at the time they make the decision to donate, but nevertheless be rewarded subsequently by a society that recognizes the value of their contributions.

Difficulties arise when donors have expectations of reward that they do not articulate, or when organ donors and recipients may conspire to disguise commercial transactions. There are also cases where organ donors are motivated to help out of concern for the welfare of the recipients but, at the same time, also entertain the possibility of having their own acute needs addressed in the process. Illustrative cases help to explain how complicated the task can be for authorities and members of transplant ethics committees when they are obliged to use a rigid and narrow understanding of altruism in order to determine which applications for organ donation are acceptable.

Extended families and the extension of altruism

Useful illustrations of the difficulties mentioned above are provided in a couple of cases.

One case involves a member of the Philippine President's Cabinet who received a transplant kidney from a chauffeur who he personally employed. In many respects, the nature of the employment was defined by their personal relationship. The chauffeur lived within the employer's household long before the need for a transplant was discovered. He was known to other members of the household as being a family insider. He shared provincial roots with the employer. He was missed by household members when absent from social gatherings.

When the chauffeur offered his kidney for transplant, it did not come as a surprise to the household members. The chauffeur said it was a good opportunity to help someone who was in great need. He did not ask for compensation but was happy later on to learn that his "employer" felt he had to take care of his family (Salaverria 2007).

This example presents a challenge to the notion of *kagandahang loob* because of, among other things, the possibility of coercion arising from the existence of an employer–employee relationship as well as from the high position of authority held by the recipient. Each of these factors can be coercive in itself, especially because the donor's situation in life can be contrasted with the recipient's elevated economic and political status. Thus, one may argue that the chauffeur's being an employee of the beneficiary could have posed undue influence on his decision-making. The chauffeur could also have been aware of material benefits that could have come his way in recognition of the kidney donation. These benefits could well have been the main factors that motivated him. If so, his offer to donate would not have been purely altruistic.

If these points were raised in a context where the benefactor and beneficiary were not part of the same household and did not share a common history, they would constitute quite strong objections. Indeed, transplant ethics committees in the Philippines have had to deal with applications for organ transplantation where the employer–employee relationship between recipient and donor could have the effect of applying coercive pressure because of the employee's lack of job security or employment alternatives. The pressures are compounded because the employees could anticipate material rewards even in situations where the recipients do not make any promises to them. In such cases, the claim to altruistic giving would be questionable.

The lack of altruism could also give rise to harmful consequences for both donor and beneficiary because, when genuine concern of each for the other is missing, important safety measures in the transplantation procedure could be sacrificed. Strictly material reciprocity between donors and recipients has been documented to lead to poor outcomes for donors (Zargooshi 2001a, 2001b; Goyal *et al.* 2002; Naqvi *et al.* 2007; Awaya *et al.* 2009; Moazam *et al.* 2009; Tong *et al.* 2012). In addition, greater risks for recipients could arise from inaccurate medical histories taken from non-altruistic donors (for example, about compromised blood transfusions they may have received).

On the other hand, the narrative above suggests a family perspective characterized by offerings and counter-offerings of *kagandahang loob*. Having probably been the recipient of *kagandahang loob* at various points in his life, the chauffeur decided that the acute medical need of his employer gave him an opportunity to respond with his own *kagandahang loob*. The relationship between donor and recipient was a pre-existing one, rather than one that was just being established. It could not be defined solely by the organ donation. Defining the relationship in that way would have disregarded the bonds built over time not only between the donor and the recipient but also among the wider membership of their community.

To further understand the nature of the relationship, one recalls the significance of *hiya* in relation to *kagandahang loob* and *utang na loob*. Even when an organ donor does not expect to be repaid, the organ recipient should feel an obligation to repay. Not to feel this obligation is to be *walang hiya*. Hence an organ recipient gets caught in a dilemma. Confronted with a transplant ethics committee investigation, organ recipients would effectively have had to pretend they did not intend to repay (and bear the burden of being *walang hiya*) so that the organ transplant could be approved.

This point needs a bit of elaboration as to what repayment may consist of. The problematic cases are those that involve poor donors whose acute and immediate needs could only be met if money or material reward were involved. The organ donor may be in dire need of a means of livelihood. An amount of money for use as capital would then be very useful. Or, he might have a son or daughter who needs hospitalization for a serious condition. He needs money to pay hospital bills. One can go back to what was mentioned above regarding the importance of the material as a vehicle for *kagandahang loob*. While recognizing the primacy of the *kalooban* (the inner self) the material benefit cannot be totally ignored. The material benefit takes on an extra-material dimension within that organ-sharing context.

There are important nuances in relationships that can be overlooked when we limit uncritically our lenses of understanding to those of prevailing paradigms. These paradigms prove to be convenient when laws or regulations are promulgated to draw the boundary between what is allowable and what is not. However, they do not necessarily capture the nuances that spell the difference between virtuous behaviour and behaviour that deserves punishment.

Not having access to the confidential minutes of the transplant ethics committee that deliberated on this first case, one can only surmise that that committee approved this living non-related organ donation because it recognized that the prevailing paradigm of altruism that required consanguinity, or the absence of any expectation of reciprocation, needed to be broadened to accommodate such situations. The Cabinet member and the chauffeur were part of an extended family whose members cared for one another and shared their inner selves as well as what they had in material terms.

The second example (based on first-hand knowledge) illustrates additional issues that arise under more controversial circumstances:

> As a young boy, Mario was involved in street fights a number of times. One of those times, the police happened to be around. They wanted to apprehend Mario because of his direct involvement. He was about to be brought to the precinct when the Village Chairman intervened and Mario was remanded in his care instead. The Village Chairman guaranteed that Mario would not be involved again in any street fights. Five years later, Mario learned that the Village Chairman was ill and needed a kidney transplant. Mario donated one of his kidneys, notwithstanding objections of his sister and mother. Although Mario did not ask for payment, the Village Chairman promised that he would give him a tricycle (a motorized bike with a sidecar to carry passengers) so he could earn a living.

On one interpretation, Mario was returning the *kagandahang loob* that he received from the Village Chairman five years earlier. The elements of *kagandahang loob* are present in this narrative. Mario acted voluntarily – without being asked. Second, he expressed his desire to make the donation before the Village Chairman said he would give him a tricycle. Hence, he became committed to the donation without expectation of that reward. Third, Mario had a genuine feeling of concern for the Chairman, whose *kagandahang loob* he recognized. Nevertheless, based on applicable regulations pertaining to organ transplantation, there are two reasons why transplantation in such circumstances would not have been allowed to proceed. The first is the lack of blood relationship between donor and recipient. The second is the presence of material reward.

The Philippine Department of Health (Secretary of Health 2010, 3) says that a living non-related donation is "permitted only when it is voluntary and truly altruistic, without any kind of compensation or gratuity package attached to it". The administrative order also says that "[p]ayment as a precondition for kidney donation and sale and purchase of kidneys by kidney vendors/commercial donors are strictly prohibited", that "kidney transplantation is not part of medical tourism" and that "foreigners are not eligible to receive organs from Filipino non-related donors" (ibid., 3). These three provisions are consistent with a *kagandahang loob* framework for understanding organ donation in that they aim to exclude opportunities for organ "donation" from those who have a primary interest in material compensation. The provisions also prohibit organ transplants to tourists and foreigners who, because of their circumstances, could not be regarded as having a previously established relationship with local organ donors.

Concerning the absence of consanguinity, one can focus on the reasoning behind the regulation that is pertinent to this chapter. A first point has to do with respect for the family's autonomy in decision-making. Organ transplantation involves risks for the donor and it is important to ensure that such risks are understood and properly evaluated in relation to benefits. When a transplant takes place among family members, the presumption seems to be that within that family, a decision can be arrived at that takes individual members' interests into account in a way that is fair and acceptable to all. It is assumed that there is an abundance of *kagandahang loob* and that decisions about addressing acute needs of members are addressed within that context. The assumption does not always hold, of course, but it is the default interpretation.

The same presumption is not easy to make when the donor and recipient do not share family ties. Hence, outside the usual context of shared family experiences, the parties involved have the burden of proving, as in this case, that the donation is altruistically motivated. Even if the Chairman only mentioned the "reward" after the decision was made by Mario, the prohibition of payment or reward would have applied. The pertinent regulatory provision does not define the time frame within which the grant of an incentive or material compensation is prohibited. Moreover, the regulation refers to the giving or receipt of the compensation or reward without regard for the motivation of either the giver or the recipient.

Thus, Philippine regulations adopt the rigid paradigm of altruism that is focused on the absence of material rewards. However, given the extended family systems that are so widespread in the country, and given that those extended families grow through offerings and counter-offerings of *kusang loob*, one can understand the perplexity of transplant ethics committee members when they are constrained to make decisions on the basis of that rigid paradigm of altruism. *Kagandahang loob* is mainly about motivation. Understandably, motivations are not easy to determine with certainty.

The authenticity of *kagandahang loob*

These cases show how establishing the authenticity of *kagandahang loob* can be very problematic when dealing with live organ donation. Two types of issues appear to stand out. One has to do with ensuring that there is no anticipation of reward on the part of the donor. A lot of attention has focused on this process, and transplant ethics committees have probably given too much time to a task for which they do not necessarily have expertise. The other has to do with ensuring the authenticity of roles and relationships that are supposed to exist between benefactor and beneficiary.

Regarding the first type of issues, a major concern is that a living organ donor is able to disguise expectations of material reward or reciprocity. The donor and the recipient can also conceal commercial transactions. These issues have to be addressed in conjunction with the second type of issues.

The second type of issues is encountered very often when patients (or, on their behalf, close kin and friends) undertake their own (rather than a prevailing distribution system's) recruitment of organ donors. Many of them have taken the initiative to seek out genetically or emotionally related possible donors. These patients feel that the authenticity of their relationship with a donor establishes the altruistic character of the organ donation.

Some claims of having relationships can easily be confirmed. On the other hand, there are those that have obviously been contrived and therefore, lack authenticity. In between, there are those cases that call for careful investigation because, while it would be wrong to encourage commercial transactions, it would also be wrong to exclude a genuine offering of *kagandahang loob* on the basis of mere suspicions or on the basis of a notion of altruism that is incompatible with concepts of justice and solidarity within a particular society.

The cases where the donor and beneficiary form part of extended families have already been mentioned as raising difficult problems. Some of the purported relationships are characterized by some kind of economic dependence that sends organ donors (and even transplant recipients themselves) on a dangerous slippery slope to exploitation. This last classification can involve people who have presented themselves for organ transplantation under scenarios such as the following:

1 Together with his apparently poor organ donor, a rich person presents himself at a private hospital for transplantation in an economically progressive country. They claim to be distant relatives.
2 Having been married for only six months, a couple come to a hospital for a kidney transplant. The male partner comes from a rich foreign country. The wife, a native of the local developing country has offered to be the organ donor.

In cases similar to the first example, some transplant ethics committees have given the benefit of the doubt to the "consenting pair", citing reasons such as medical urgency, patient and donor autonomy, or the impracticality of verifying claims of consanguinity because the records are only available in the country of origin. One wonders why the first of these reasons could have been accepted considering that medical urgency would have made it inadvisable for the couple to travel from another country in the first place. As for the latter two reasons, their acceptance would lead us to the untenable position that almost every application for organ donation would have to be allowed among "consenting pairs" because those reasons could be invoked almost at will.

A *kagandahang loob* approach would look for a pre-existing historical relationship before authorizing organ transplantation. As the burden of proof lies with the presenting patients, the transplant ethics committee does not need to feel pressured to allow the surgery to proceed. The interests of both donor and recipient would be better served if the evaluation were done within the patients' own country. The evaluation team would then have better access to documents and to witnesses who can help to establish the existence (or non-existence) of historical bonds consistent with *kagandahang loob.*

The second case presents a situation where, ordinarily, the marriage would indicate a presumption of *kagandahang loob.* However, considering reports that Filipinas have presented themselves as kidney or liver donors too soon after getting married to foreigners, transplant ethics committees have had to be more careful. To address related issues, some transplant ethics committees and regulators have imposed minimum requirements for length of marriage before spouses could be allowed to donate organs to their partners. In general, what is needed is a delicate balancing act that seeks to ensure that such donors are truly sharing in the spirit of *kagandahang loob* and are not being exploited because of their economic dependence.

Understanding *kagandahang loob* in a comparative context

Thus far, this chapter has presented *kagandahang loob* and the related family of concepts in their interrelatedness without having to explain them indirectly in terms of seemingly equivalent concepts from classic literature that readers may be more familiar with. Comparative references could have the effect of incorrectly reducing *kagandahang loob*, for example, into the concepts that may correspond to the roughly equivalent English terms and effectively distort understanding. Nevertheless, some comparisons are useful for the purpose of bringing out a more nuanced picture of the interrelated concepts. This can be done by showing what they may be confused with in order to explain what they are not.

It is useful to compare and contrast these concepts with Mauss' observation concerning a feature of Maori law:

> the legal tie, a tie occurring through things, is one between souls, because the thing itself possesses a soul, is of the soul. Hence, it follows that to make a gift of something to someone is to make a present of some part of oneself.
>
> (Mauss 1990, 16)

In the case of *kagandahang loob*, it would be inaccurate to speak of possession of a soul, especially if the latter is taken to mean something spiritual. In Filipino discourse concerning *kagandahang loob* and *utang na loob*, there is no reference to a spiritual soul that may be found in the gift itself. Nevertheless, "making a present of some part of oneself" captures the idea of making a present of one's *kalooban* (inner self).

Related to this is the interpretation of the view regarding repayment of gifts among the Maoris that

> one clearly and logically realizes that one must give back to another person what is really part and parcel of his nature and substance, because to accept something from somebody is to accept some part of his spiritual essence, of his soul …

and not to repay "would be dangerous and mortal" because that thing coming from the person giving "exert[s] a magical or religious hold over you" (ibid., 16).

One reaction to this account in the *Essai sur le don* (*The Gift*) observes that "Mauss strives to reconstruct a whole out of parts" but realizes that that is not possible so "he has to add to the mixture an additional quantity which gives him the illusion of squaring his account" and "that quantity is *hau*" – the spirit or power in the thing given that forces the receiver to make a return (Levi-Strauss 1987, 47). This charge of "mystification" acquires greater relevance in contrasting Mauss' interpretation of the Maoris with the account given here of *kagandahang loob* because there is no room in the latter for anything spiritual or transcendent beyond the individual *kalooban*. The *kalooban* is regarded as a component of the self but not as a transcendent spirit that attaches to offerings and seeks to return to the original giver. The explanation for the obligation to give back the *utang na loob* is found in the intensity of the *hiya*, which relates to societal expectations. In local discourse, there is no suggestion of anything beyond the *hiya* to support the idea of something similar to the *hau*.

Notwithstanding these differences, one cannot discount the importance of Mauss' observations in helping to understand *utang na loob*. Aside from yielding a basic explanation for the form of contract among Polynesian clans (Mauss 1990, 16–17), Mauss' theory of the three obligations (Mauss 1990, 50) provides a useful comparative lens for viewing the *utang na loob* family of concepts. The obligation to give, to receive and to reciprocate powerfully reinforces the interplay between *kagandahang loob, utang na loob* and *hiya* in the Filipino world view. Nevertheless, one still has to exercise diligence in finding where there are differences and significant nuances that render each system unique.

Having argued in favour of accommodating transplant situations where organ donors are compensated in a way that is consistent with their social and cultural context, this chapter accepts that *utang na loob* is liable to being abused and exploited. This point is highlighted by Godelier:

> The act of giving seems to create simultaneously a twofold relationship between giver and receiver. A relationship of *solidarity* because the giver shares what he has, or what he is, with the receiver; and a relationship of *superiority* because the one who receives the gift and accepts it places

> himself in the debt of the one who has given it, thereby becoming indebted to the giver and to a certain extent becoming his "dependant", at least for as long as he has not "given back" what he was given.
>
> (Godelier 1999, 12)

An unscrupulous benefactor can take advantage of an established relationship of superiority to pressure someone with *utang na loob* to repay in a prescribed way. Out of *hiya*, that person can be "blackmailed" into a situation of submission rather than an ethically acceptable recognition of *utang na loob*. The situation could be characterized further in this way:

> Giving thus seems to establish the difference and an inequality of status between donor and recipient, which can in certain circumstances become a hierarchy: if this hierarchy already exists, then the gift expresses and legitimizes it. Two opposite movements are thus contained in a single act. The gift decreases the distance between the protagonists because it is a form of sharing, and it increases the social distance between them because one is now indebted to the other.
>
> (Godelier 1999, 12)

When wide economic disparity exists among members of a community or of an extended family, offerings and counter-offerings of *kagandahang loob* and *utang na loob* are liable to accentuate the social superiority of the economically empowered over the ones who have a limited access to economic opportunities. The superiority can be exploited, for example, by offers of compensation for transplant organs that poorer members of the community or extended family might find irresistible. An economically underprivileged member of an *utang na loob–kagandahang loob* family is liable to exploitation by an economically progressive member who is able to implant *utang na loob* with a view to extracting desired payment later. In order to address these possibilities, society needs to step in, possibly through highly capable transplant ethics committees supported by social workers and a health care team that is unencumbered by conflicts of interest.

Summary and conclusions

Organ donation deserves recognition as an act of sharing that acquires importance within a conceptual framework that may vary across different communities, cultures or countries. Its meaning and significance are defined in relation to a web of *kagandahang loob, utang na loob* and *hiya*. Within that web, the understanding of gifts, charity, reciprocity and altruism needs to be qualified by nuances relating to the interplay of the above-named concepts.

These nuances have implications for the ethical acceptability of organ transplantation that are not dependent solely on a prevailing paradigm of altruism. A paradigm that focuses on the provision (or not) of compensation for transplantable organs has gained currency because of global efforts to curb organ commodification and commercialization, human trafficking and ethically dubious types of medical tourism. While the developments appear to have resulted so far in slowing down the proliferation of the global trade, these have not been as effective within particular countries. In the Philippines, commercial transplants to foreigners appear to have been completely halted but there is no evidence of actual impact on commercial transplantation among locals (cf. de Castro 2013).

In any case, there are good reasons to propose that the evaluation of applications for transplants among non-relatives be made on the basis of guidelines and ethics evaluation protocols taking into account the framework of *kagandahang loob, utang na loob* and *hiya* as here discussed. In practical terms, this would involve the following, among other things:

First, the reorientation of transplant ethics committees away from a strict and rigid no-compensation–altruism paradigm and towards a *kagandahang loob* paradigm. The hope is that this will encourage them to be more discerning of differences in motivations among living organ donors.

Second, a serious effort to establish and implement protocols for determining authenticity of *kagandahang loob.* This would have to be done by a health care team that included professionals and social workers trained for the purpose.

Third, formulation of a system to mediate acceptable forms of *utang na loob* repayment or reciprocation by transplant organ beneficiaries. This is needed to enable the beneficiaries to transcend the *hiya* that pushes them to compensate their organ donors.

Fourth, provision of assistance to organ donors who may be liable to exploitation so they can be shown that there are ways for them to earn money by rechannelling their *kagandahang loob.*

While some transplant ethics committees have carried out tasks assigned to them faithfully and in accordance with international guidelines, there has to be room for flexibility to the extent that variation can be justified. One can also remove the basis for the perplexity that sometimes overcomes a transplant ethics committee when it sees a mis-fit between local cultural concepts and the recommended manner of implementing some globally accepted guidelines. We should be able to justify some variation in implementation on the basis of *kagandahang loob, utang na loob* and *hiya* without sacrificing general ethical principles.

References

Awaya, T., Siruno, L., Toledano, S.J., Aguilar, F., Shimazono, Y., and L.D. de Castro. 2009. "Failure of Informed Consent in Compensated Non-Related Kidney Donation in the Philippines." *Asian Bioethics Review* 1–2: 138–143.

Befu, H. 1977. "Social Exchange." *Annual Review of Anthropology* 6: 255–281.

Bulatao, J.C. 1964. "Hiya." *Philippine Studies* 12: 424–428.

de Castro, L.D. 1998. "Debts of Good Will and Interpersonal Justice." Proceedings of the Twentieth World Congress of Philosophy, 10–15 August 1998. Boston University. Available at: www.bu.edu/wcp/Papers/Asia/AsiaDeCa.htm.

de Castro, L.D. 2013. "The Declaration of Istanbul in the Philippines: Success with Foreigners but a Continuing Challenge for Local Transplant Tourism." *Medicine, Health Care and Philosophy* 16: 929–932.

Godelier, M. 1999. *The Enigma of the Gift*. Translated by Nora Scott. Oxford: Blackwell Publishers.

Goyal, M., Mehta, R.L., Schneiderman, L.J., and A.R. Sehgal. 2002. "Economic and Health Consequences of Selling a Kidney in India." *Journal of American Medical Association* 288: 1589–1593.

Hollnsteiner, M. 1973. "Reciprocity in the Lowland Philippines." In: *Four Readings on Philippine Values. IPC 2*, edited by F. Lynch and A. de Guzman, 69–92. Quezon City: Ateneo de Manila University Press.

Kaut, C. 1961. "*Utang na loob*: A System of Contractual Obligation among Tagalog." *Southwestern Journal of Anthropology* 17: 256–272.

Levi-Strauss, C. 1987. *Introduction to the Work of Marcel Mauss*. London: Routledge.

Lynch, F. 1962. "Philippine Values II: Social Acceptance." *Philippine Studies* 10(1): 82–99.

Mauss, M. 1990. *The Gift*. Translated by W. D. Halls. Oxford: Routledge.

Moazam, F., Zaman, R.M., and A.M. Jafarey. 2009. "Conversations with Kidney Vendors in Pakistan." *Asian Bioethics Review* 1–2: 108–137.

Naqvi, S.A.A., Ali, B., Mazhar, F., Zafar, M.N., and S.A.A. Rizvi. 2007. "A Socio-economic Survey of Kidney Vendors in Pakistan." *Transplant International* 20(11): 934–939.

Panopio, I.S., and R.S. Rolda. 2006. *Society and Culture: Introduction to Sociology and Anthropology*. Quezon City: Katha Publishing Co., Inc.

Participants in the International Summit on Transplant Tourism and Organ Trafficking. 2008. "The Declaration of Istanbul on Organ Trafficking and Transplant Tourism." *Kidney International* 74: 854–859.

Quisumbing, L.R. 1976. "Filipino Social Values and Attitudes in Relation to Development." In: *Changing Identities in Modern Southeast Asia*, edited by D.J. Banks, 256–268. The Hague: Mouton and Co.

Salaverria, L. 2007. "It Feels Good to Help – Gonzalez's Kidney Donor." *The Philippine Daily Inquirer*. Available at: http://newsinfo.inquirer.net/breakingnews/metro/view_article.php?article_id=89345.

Secretary of Health. 2010. Administrative Order 2010–0018.

Tong, A., Chapman, J.R., Wong, G., Cross, N.B., Batabyal, P., and J.C. Craig. 2012. "The Experiences of Commercial Kidney Donors: Thematic Synthesis of Qualitative Research." *Transplant International* 25(11): 1138–1149.

WHO (World Health Organization). 2010. "Guiding Principles on Human Cell, Tissue and Organ Transplantation." *Transplantation* 90: 229.

WMA (World Medical Association General Assembly). 2014. WMA Statement on Human Organ Donation and Transplantation. Available at: www.wma.net/en/30publications/10policies/20archives/t7.

Zargooshi, J. 2001a. "Iranian Kidney Donors: Motivations and Relations with Recipients." *Journal of Urology* 165(2): 386–392.

Zargooshi, J. 2001b. "Quality of Life of Iranian Kidney Donors." *Journal of Urology* 166(5): 1790–1799.

6 Sharing amidst scarcity

The commons as innovative transgression in xeno- and allotransplant science

Lesley A. Sharp

Introduction

Sharing is by nature a social act. As a verb, in (American) English, "to share" imparts several meanings: to divide among two or more parties, where each takes a part; to enjoy something with others; to have something in common with others; and to portion out something in one's possession that others might enjoy, desire or require. "To share" necessitates giving up something, and so the act itself imparts sacrifice and harbours sentimental qualities and possibilities. Sharing connotes kindness and trust, and it can suspend or circumvent boundaries of social difference: one shares goods, possessions, food, social space or information and, in so doing, one diffuses disparities (we share so that others are not excluded), or brings others into the realm of sociality (sharing with others engenders or strengthens bonds of friendship and kinship). Because sharing may involve partitioning things into equal portions, sharing may serve (albeit temporarily) as a social equalizer: as the act of sharing proclaims, we may be different in other contexts, but when we share we temporarily become social equivalents of one another. To share unequally, on the other hand, is to withhold, to be miserly and, in so doing, one reaffirms social hierarchies.

If, as Mauss asserted long ago, gift-giving is an intricate social process (Mauss 1967), sharing defines a specialized or more rarefied form of gifting, one that relies on a delicate calculus of giving because one must consider what, and how much, to distribute, and whether the goods, or social space, or services, or sentiments portioned out are fleeting or permanent; what and how much one should give away; and whether one should merely loan to those in need. As such, sharing is a temporalized social act, because one might expect that which was given would later be returned. (Indeed, in many American contexts, when one asks politely to "borrow" something, one is really asking permission to "share" with no intention of return.)

These qualities – *sentimentality, scarcity* and *temporality* – frame this chapter. My overall goals are as follows: to examine, first, what differentiates sharing from gift-giving; second, how scarcity might initiate sharing; and, third, how sharing, as a social, temporalized process, generates unusual, innovative, and, even, subversive acts. I situate my arguments within two interrelated medical contexts: *allotransplantation* (or what I prefer to call *human organ transfer*), which involves the salvaging of reusable organ(s) from one human body (a living or deceased "donor") for subsequent (re)use in one or several sickly patient(s) (or "recipient(s)"); and *xenotransplantation* (henceforth *xeno*), a highly experimental realm of transplant research intent on culling organs from various animal species for human use. A range of animals have figured as potential "source" or "donor" species in xeno research, most notably non-human primates (especially baboons and chimpanzees) and, since the 1990s, transgenic pigs whose genome is partially human. Whereas allotransplantation has proved extraordinarily successful, thanks to the development of potent immunosuppressants, xeno science has faltered repeatedly as a promising experimental alternative because of extraordinarily challenging transpecies immunological hurdles that current drug regimens are unable to overcome. Sharing surfaces within each domain as an unmarked yet remarkable social practice. Taking a comparative approach I explore how scarcity initiates sharing within each; I ask how we might differentiate the social consequences of gift-giving versus sharing; and I consider how allo- and xenotransplant science together inform alternative readings of sharing's potential as both a temporalized and subversive social act. My analysis is framed by my interest in the sociomoral consequences of sharing in the broader realm of organ transplant surgery and research (Sharp 2013).

Sharing and sociality in medical science

Acts of sharing may be driven by scarcity, a reality made all too clear as we shift our attention to healthcare domains. In acute as well as chronically overtaxed, undersupplied and poorly funded contexts, healthcare personnel must make do with what they have at hand. Nurses, surgeons, technicians and the like might draw on sharing as an innovative practice: they might wash and reuse disposable technologies and tools, or require that patients share rooms or, even, beds. Patients, too, may resort to sharing as an innovative survival strategy: to assist the destitute, they might stockpile and redistribute surplus medications to strangers, acquaintances and friends (Sharp 2002; Wendland 2010; Livingston 2012).

The national organization that oversees the fair distribution of donated organs within the US is UNOS, or the United Network for Organ *Sharing*; yet, interestingly, "sharing" is not a favoured term within the UNOS lexicon and among transplant professionals nationwide. Instead, all involved parties are trained early on to speak instead of organ "donation" and of organs as "gifts", terms that convert bodies and their parts into inert, albeit precious, things that point to different sorts of fleeting sociality. Where specifically cadaveric donation is concerned (involving donors who most often have been declared brain dead) (Sharp 2006b), one permanently and anonymously gives organs and tissue to others in need with neither any intent or hope of retrieval, nor knowledge of who these parties might be. Body parts, as gifts, move in one direction only and, once given away, they become the inalienable parts – and possessions – of *other* people, the majority of whom will always remain strangers to their respective gift-givers. Within the US especially, this sort of rhetorical policing (Richardson 1996) of self and others delineates clear boundaries between appropriate and taboo ways to speak of and think about organ transfer (Sharp 2001). In turn, rhetorical policing regularly figures in debates among social scientists, clinicians, bioethicists and transplant specialists over when and whether donors' bodies are or should be commodified (Murray 1987; Sells 1992; Nelkin and Andrews 1998; Rothman *et al.* 1997; Jackson 2002; Scheper-Hughes and Wacquant 2003; Waldby and Mitchell 2006). The rhetoric of donation itself generates paradoxical circumstances that undermine the values associated with sociality by insisting that organs are gifts that, nevertheless, cannot be repaid or reciprocated, a reality that Siminoff and Chillag have referred to as "the fallacy of the 'gift of life'" (Siminoff and Chillag 1999).

Organ "donation", then, involves a series of complex acts and an associated reframing of how one should think about bodies and their parts. In cases involving cadaveric donation, one must simultaneously embrace unusual categories of death (including brain death and cardiac arrest without resuscitation) that then facilitate the mining of bodies for their reusable, lifesaving potential. Living donors in turn must, quite literally, give of themselves to assist others, decisions that involve not only great acts of kindness and sacrifice, but a willingness to consider parts of their bodies as redundant (because one can give away one of a pair of lungs, kidneys or, even, corneas, or segments of one's liver). As my ethnographic data reveal, the performative acts and private sentiments of such involved lay parties as donors, recipients and their respective kin expose a widespread tendency to challenge professional understandings of organ transfer. I assert that whereas professionals promote donations as permanent acts of loss and renewal, lay parties readily understand the same processes not merely as the giving away, but as the *sharing* of a donor's body parts *and* vitality. As a result, the process of sharing facilitates a merging of selves. Sharing in these contexts – far more so than in persistently anonymous donations – engenders eclectic and unusual forms of sociality among donors, recipients, and their respective kin; furthermore, sharing provokes long-term and richly affective responses, too.

Here I wish to probe the sociomoral consequences of this shift in registers from "donation" to "sharing" within the overlapping realms of allo- and xenotransplantation. I employ a looping effect (Hacking 1995) of sorts, where attention to muted, misunderstood and forbidden lay sentiments about allotransplants-as-sharing helps uncover still other innovative forms of sharing within xeno research, where involved scientists sometimes share animal stock – generating what I reference as an "animal commons" – when faced with research failures and the evacuation of research funds. These developments within xeno science embolden me to return yet again at this chapter's conclusion to allotransplantation to propose the radical possibility of a *human* commons.

The sentimental structures of scarcity, experimental failure and biocapital

The arguments posed throughout this chapter are informed by a set of over-arching premises. First, donation rhetoric, alongside the affective dimensions of sharing, is informed by widespread anxieties over organ scarcity. Scarcity is frequently regarded in transplant circles as a stark and inescapable reality that complicates a specialized field of biomedicine plagued by potentially irresolvable conflicts over whether transferred body parts should be acquired through Samaritan acts of kindness, or should be commodified (generally within regulated markets) to increase their supply. Second, xeno researchers, determined to generate highly experimental alternatives to the human organ supply, are similarly driven by anxieties over chronic organ shortages nationally and globally (Sharp 2013). Third, xeno scientists' persistent determination, even in the face of repeated failures, is fuelled by xeno's social and economic promissory qualities (Franklin and Lock 2003; Guyer 2007), informed, on the one hand, by the ethos of a humanitarian desire to relieve human suffering (Sharp 2013) and lured, on the other, by the lucrative promises of futuristic biocapital (Rose 2001; Sunder Rajan 2006; Cooper 2008). Fourth, xeno science proffers an especially "lively" example of biocapital (Sunder Rajan 2012), where involved experts hope to "humanize" (Cooper and Lanza 2000) living things – and, in this instance, pigs – through genetic manipulation so as to mine these animals' bodies as alternative sources for human body repair. Fifth, a heavy reliance on public and private investors sustains ongoing (and consistently faltering) research in xeno research, and this generates its own set of anxieties. Innovative scientists and inventors are well aware of the fickleness of venture capital, whose actors frequently demand rapid research results and financial returns, paired with very real threats of the evacuation of sustaining capital. As a realm of science marked consistently by significant immunological challenges, decades of failed transpecies surgeries and a sluggish rate of progress, xeno science struggles to retain steady support.

In response to these factors, however, xeno scientists have not abandoned their pursuits. Rather, such challenges have engendered innovations designed to sustain lab activities and ensure the integrity of lab animal colonies. While scientists wait out the hiatus in financial support, some cut corners (and potentially compromise research) by, for instance, piggybacking on other well-funded projects or by employing the same animal in multiple experiments. Others have turned their attention to new projects in the hopes that the current funding drought affecting xeno is only temporary, leaving their work in a state of suspended animation. Still others offer evidence of an emergent animal commons, where prized hybrid animals are shared among previously competing scientists and their associated labs. With these premises in mind, this chapter is best understood as a preliminary effort to explore the significance of the animal commons as an innovative strategy of scientific survival, one that bears the potential of looping back and informing readings of other sharing strategies encountered within allotransplantation.

Organ transfer: sharing amid scarcity

Sharing, as a laudatory social practice, defines a dominant, albeit informal and, even, underground discourse within the clinical realm of human-to-human organ transfer. Though pervasive within lay circles, even there its specific meanings are murky. In the US, one regularly encounters professionals' descriptions of organ transfer as "donations", "gifts", "lifesaving" and "heroic" acts, but generally not specifically as acts of "sharing". Although not widely encouraged by transplant professionals (some of whom may even strive to forbid it), living donors (or deceased donors' kin) and organ recipients increasingly reach out to communicate with or meet one another (Sharp 2001, 2007).

Tracking acts of sociality within this surgical realm is tricky and necessitates systematic and long-term ethnographic attention. Among the most problematic aspects of organ transfer is that official rhetoric and associated sanctioned practices, as promoted by transplant professionals, contradict (and, thus, officially condemn) the peculiar twists and turns that define an inevitable part of the lived experiences of involved lay parties, most notably transplant recipients and the surviving kin of deceased organ donors. Written exchanges and personal encounters rapidly develop into reciprocal relationships, often marked, first, by the exchange of anonymous cards and letters, which may then fuel desires to meet in person. During initial phases, personal exchanges and encounters are bureaucratically orchestrated by transplant professionals who insist on guarding the anonymity of all involved parties. Once face-to-face encounters occur, the power of the organ as "gift" engenders strong, interpersonal bonds most often glossed by involved lay parties as those of kinship, replete with expressions of both love and obligation (Sharp 2006b).

I believe that these exchanges, and subsequent forms of sociality, are driven not merely by the idea that organs are precious "gifts" (as professionals insist), but that body parts harbour the essence of their donors, and that both qualities render the organ as something unique and precious that is not simply given away or "gifted" but *shared* across the donor–recipient divide. That is, the initial partitioning of the body, so that its organs may be shared with others, produces unique and innovative forms of sociality. These include acts of commensality (such as sharing holidays, birthdays and Sunday meals), the giving of still other special gifts endowed with personal or historical significance (including mementos from a deceased donor's life, or the making of memorial quilts) and occupying prominent roles during key ritual moments, including baptisms, weddings and funerals. As organ recipients often remark, they are forever indebted, often "for life", to their donors or donors' kin, and such sentiments encourage a range of involved lay parties to open up and share their lives with others in ways that would have seemed unimaginable before their surgeries (for an interesting comparison see Heinemann 2014).

Communication between the surviving kin of deceased donors and transplant recipients has long been viewed as transgressive, and many professions have sought actively to prohibit or control letter writing and face-to-face encounters, fearing such correspondence would undermine a patient's ability to heal physically and psychologically, based on an assumption that mourning renders donor kin emotionally unstable and, even, potentially dangerous. Numerous professionals have spoken to me of their fears that donor kin might even physically attack a transplant recipient, whose body now harbours an organ of their deceased loved one, or that they would seek out financial reparations for their "gifts". (I have yet to encounter a story of any such event occurring.) In short, they fear that donor kin might reclaim their rights to parts they once gave away to another. Such fears spring, I believe, from a misunderstanding of how lay parties understand organ donation not merely as donations, but as acts of sharing. Whereas professionals fear that donor kin might secretly view donated organs as precious commodities (and thus as bearing promises of financial gain), donor kin and recipients who seek out one another might do so because of their "shared" understanding of "sharing" as a natural social process activated by organ transfer. Thus, whereas professionals are troubled by the consequences of viewing organs as anything but private property – once released from their natal bodies, they now belong to those in whom they have been surgically transplanted – involved lay parties understand that such "goods" possess unique or "singular" qualities and, further, that they are imbued with social lives (Kopytoff 1986) that spring from mutual understandings of what sharing entails.

Lay parties thus express very different understandings of the ethos of giving, and central to this is the sense that a donated organ remains a special sort of living thing, or a vital part of something, or, more often, someone now dead and lost. Within this alternative framework, parts simply cannot be discarded, or merely given away or donated to strangers in need (like a bag of now ill-fitting clothes). Instead, they are *shared* things that naturally insist upon newly established forms of sociality. Donor kin offer something very precious to others, and, in so doing, they understand that they are transferring the care of the lost loved one to strangers who are simultaneously in need of repair. In response, such strangers might later be integrated as newfound, beloved kin. Thus, whereas professionals most readily view donation as a one-way transfer (while nevertheless employing the language of gift-giving to encourage lay participation), they may struggle in private with the possibility that organs are in fact forms of "lively [bio]capital" (Sunder Rajan 2006, 2012). Together, many donor kin and organ recipients find the weight – or what Fox and Swazey long ago identified so astutely as the potential "tyranny" – of so powerful a gift (Fox and Swazey 1992) as instilling, initiating, and, even, necessitating long-term forms of sharing of one's life with newfound others.

As such contradictory responses reveal, transferred human organs are understood by different parties as either inert (and potentially commodified) or as living things. Rendered as inert within the professional realm, an organ's reification is palpable: professionals – be they surgeons, nurses or social workers – generally balk at the idea that a human organ, retrieved from a brain-dead human being, could harbour the life essence, spirit, soul, history or memories of the dead. Within the surgeon's realm, an organ is understood as a replaceable part devoid of a past, or personalized history. This is especially evident during those moments when professionals speak to organ recipients about where their organs came from: details provided are generally limited to the sex and age of the deceased donor, alongside vague geographical references (the region of the country or state where the deceased donor resided, without naming counties, towns or neighbourhoods), and only sometimes will they provide the cause of death (and usually only if it did not involve a homicide or suicide). This economizing of details is a deliberate temporal exercise, one that allows recipients to generate new histories, past and future, of their own without having to bear the emotional weight of their donors' pasts.

When donor kin and recipients correspond by letter or meet in person, however, organs are rapidly reanimated as living things that harbour elaborate pasts. The sharing of the life stories of the dead fosters a strong sense of joint obligation to care for the precious organ (by caring for oneself), and to embrace others, who were once strangers, as members of the intricate web of one's personal life. As I describe elsewhere, among the most profound revelations is the widespread understanding that through organ transplantation one now has two mothers – one's own birth mother and, now, one's "donor mother" for whom one may well perform filial duties previously shouldered by a deceased donor at those times when the donor mother is in need (see Sharp 2006b).

As this discussion illustrates, "sharing" operates on several registers at once. Where the organ becomes thingified, it involves the transfer, and, thus, the sharing of precious, medicalized goods. Objectified as such, transferred organs are most certainly commodified: their preciousness is reflected in their price tags (organ transplants for hearts and livers can run in the US$100,000s), accumulating worth – and associated costs – as they emerge at the site of the procurement surgery, travel by plane or helicopter in the hands of transplant professionals, and then make their way to yet another surgical theatre to be implanted in the prepped body of the recipient (whose excised natal organ is deemed of little use and is discarded as medical waste). The worth assigned to these body-parts-as-goods is inescapably determined by their scarcity. As reiterated in all transplant literature, public forums and during professional conference presentations, the number of potential recipients awaiting organs far surpasses those of donated organs, a paired set of progressions of Malthusian proportions.

Scarcity, then, is the sociomoral lynchpin of the troubled ethical world of allotransplantation. Were scarcity not an issue, one might well anticipate that professionals would no longer so strictly and vigilantly police communication across the donor/recipient divide. (Currently, they do so in large part out of fear of bad publicity – after all, stories of demanding donor kin could derail the fragile economy in donated body parts.) Scarcity also drives the never-ending, periodic revival of proposals to commercialize the supply of organs (by offering money or other incentives to donor kin willing to consent to the procurement of organs from deceased relatives), an approach that, needless to say, existing donor kin find abhorrent because such proposals debase their own acts of selflessness, kindness, sacrifice and love, all of which define the very core of post-surgical sharing.

Xeno research and the science of scarcity

As we shift our attention to highly experimental realms of transplant research, it soon becomes clear that involved scientists' efforts likewise are driven in large part by anxieties surrounding chronic organ scarcity. Xeno scientists, for instance, are intent on producing alternatives to allografting in the hopes of one day eliminating altogether the surgical dependence on human organ donors. I often think of xeno and other experimental researchers (in the field of bioengineering) as driven by a "what if" sort of logic: what if any and all failing solid organs could be swopped out for parts of non-human origin? New organs could be cultured and then grown ex-vivo in "source animals" so as to be tailor-made for individual patients. Animals – ranging from non-human primates to, more recently, genetically altered pigs – could be raised as "donor species" whose fleshy parts could replace ailing ones in human patients. The experimental imaginary (Sharp 2013) of xeno research circulates at the outermost boundary where scarcity and imagined possibilities coexist, a domain plagued by ongoing failure yet nevertheless focused on the hope and hype of future possibilities in the *longue durée* (Sunder Rajan 2006; Guyer 2007; Cooper 2008).

Amidst this entangled set of challenges, xeno researchers are faced with scarcity of another sort: namely, the rather sudden evacuation of investment capital. Xeno research involves a wide swath of researchers, including immunologists, research veterinarians and surgeons, all of whom are intent on discovering ways in which to fool the human immune system into perceiving tissue derived from another species as "self" rather than "other". To claim that the immunological hurdles are challenging is an understatement. Human bodies readily and rapidly recognize tissue derived from other humans as foreign (consider, for instance, the importance of blood typing before initiating a transfusion), and, unless fully inert (as with processed bone), implanted parts derived from animals immediately initiate a cascade of life-threatening hyper-acute immunological responses.

Throughout the twentieth century, xeno scientists have tinkered with a range of animal species, eventually embracing by mid-century non-human primates (especially baboons and chimps) who are regarded as being our closest evolutionary "cousins", as our best immunological matches (Eagle 1963; Fletcher *et al.* 1986; Starzl *et al.* 1993; *Nature* 1984; Cooper and Lanza 2000; Sharp 2006a). The use of simian species was nevertheless plagued by financial woes (because primates are difficult to obtain and very expensive to maintain), alongside growing public protest and activist outrage over their use as laboratory subjects (Donnelley 1999a, 1999b; Corbey 2005). In the end, a preference for primates gave way to the now current practice of cultivating transgenic swine as an emergent "source" animal or "donor" species (*Lancet* 1997; Calne 1997, 2005; de Burgh 1998; Butler 2002; Kaebnick 2002; Lemonick 2002; Cook 2006).

Within xeno science, pigs are now celebrated as a far more viable alternative to primates for several reasons: they are widely regarded in science as anatomically similar to humans; they mature quickly and produce large litters; they can be selectively bred for size and other characteristics with ease over only a few generations; because they are classified as farm, rather than laboratory, animals, they are much cheaper to obtain and maintain; and as an already ubiquitous food source, they are widely regarded as industrially farmed "utilitarian" animals that generate far fewer emotionally heated responses among the lay public than do primates.

Although xeno research has most certainly faced a range of immunological challenges, no blow hit harder than the threat of zoonotic infections that could cross the species barrier undetected at the molecular level. The scourge of xeno science is PERVs, or porcine endogenous retroviruses, often described in lay terms as "porcine AIDS", an endemic infection uncovered in the 1990s and now understood as so endemic to the species as to be integrated into the genome of pigs worldwide (Patience *et al.* 1997; Weiss 1998; Sypniewski *et al.* 2005). PERVs, alongside repeated failures to overcome hyper-acute immunological rejection, rapidly shifted xeno research from being the darling to being the pariah of venture capital (Maeder and Ross 2002). Intriguingly, within xeno science, this common farm animal now figures prominently in a newly imagined form of animal commons.

Pigs and the animal commons

Cutting edge, highly experimental research, in the US at least, inevitably generates proprietary knowledge. During presentations at scientific conferences, for instance, researchers from diverse fields of biotech frequently stop short of providing all supporting data and, when asked by the audience to clarify their findings, it is not unusual to hear presenters claim that they can speak no further because of "trade secrets" and "proprietary knowledge". The lucrative qualities of biotech (and associated biocapital, such as transgenic swine) hinge in large part on acquiring patents on technologies, procedures, engineered genes and cell lines and associated specialized knowledge. This is true even where academic research projects in the US are concerned, given the long-standing presence of the private sector on the campuses of research universities, alongside the propensity among scientists today to establish off-campus, private, "spin-off" companies to protect their findings from their universities' attempts to claim ownership. These sorts of developments occur within xeno science, although I have found this to be relatively muted in contrast to other domains (such as artificial organ design in bioengineering). I suspect this springs from the fact that bioengineers are trained in a field that has a long history of "applied" work where the goal is to produce marketable products, whereas xeno experts tend to be academic immunologists and surgical researchers most interested in what they describe as "pure" science.

Xeno science nevertheless must bridge academic and market spheres because of its heavy reliance on venture capital derived from individual, private investors and from pharmaceutical corporations, all of whom hope to profit from the promissory nature of pigs. Sadly, however, both investment sources rapidly withdrew support when xeno experiments proved an abysmal failure (Sharp 2013) and were threatened, too, by the imagined epi- and, even, pandemic threat of PERVs (Sharp 2014). Rather than abandoning the field, however, a handful of leading xeno experts based in five separate Anglophone countries (the US, the UK, Canada, New Zealand and Australia) made a radical decision: they established, for all intents and purposes, an animal commons of porcine "source" herds.

To explain how this came about I must backtrack for a moment. Over the course of the last three decades or so, xeno experts have reached the conclusion that if pigs are to prove feasible as organ "donor" species, they must be transformed genetically. Strategies currently assume a range of forms, most notably involving attempts to "knock out" proteins, etc., inherent in pigs that the human immune system would otherwise recognize and attack as "not human/not self"; and parallel efforts to "humanize" pigs and transform them into immunological "chimeras" whose genome incorporates transpecies genetic material (First and Haseltine 1988; Cooper and Lanza 2000; d'Apice *et al.* 2001). In lay terminology, decades of innovative research has produced specialized herds of genetically modified or "engineered" animals bred for immunologically relevant traits, size and still other key qualities, and maintained in isolation on farms tied to leading xeno laboratories. Indeed, in one instance I encountered a world-renowned xeno expert who had withdrawn from cutting edge lab research to devote himself fulltime to overseeing a specialized prized herd of transgenic pigs. Whereas in many quarters of science entire colonies of animals are euthanized when the funding runs dry or public protests mount (shifting a lab's investments to cold storage in order to maintain frozen embryos and semen, see for instance Pollack 2012), xeno experts view their living swine as too precious to sacrifice when faced with the evacuation of investment capital. In response, leaders in the field have opted not only to preserve living swine, but to share proprietary knowledge by supplying one another with prized animals from their own herds.

Xeno's animal commons emerges as a radical and innovative form of professional sharing, proposed in the face of scarcity brought on by the evacuation of investment capital. Animals derived from herds once understood as the private property of individual labs are now transported and shared across state and international boundaries. When I expressed incredulity when I first learned of this practice, one scientist explained that sharing animals with other labs helped to ensure progress within the field for all. Sharing, in this context, took several forms, including farming out gilts to other national labs, and shipping frozen embryos or boar semen to those based abroad. The potential to generate breakthrough knowledge means that in the end a single lab could profit from the efforts of others, whose staff would in turn share their knowledge with the original developer because they had all been active participants in the animal commons of xeno science.

In writing of such practices elsewhere, Hyde defines the notion of the commons as a "right of action" involving property that is held collectively, and where such rights are "bundled together" so that "no part can be split off as a separable property" (Hyde 2010, 24–27, 40–41). Hyde's description of the (original) agrarian commons (after Thompson 1993) seems eerily prescient of xeno's animal commons: as Hyde (2010, 43) explains, members "are not individuals in the free market sense but a species, rather, of public or collective being". Within the context I describe involving xeno science, we might well read associated "species" as being both human and porcine. Practices within xeno offer little evidence thus far of a true or "endurable" (ibid., 43–44) commons, however. This shortcoming rests on xeno's animal commons' tentativeness and the risky hopes of its longevity. One might predict, for instance, that the animal commons could quickly collapse if and when a renewed injection of investment capital lures what Hyde calls "self-interested individuals" (ibid., 44) away from the collective. In the meantime, the animal commons offers an intriguing example of sharing amid scarcity so that the science itself can avoid faltering and, instead, remain in a holding pattern of sorts. Within this rarefied domain of science, not only are animals themselves a "shared resource", but they figure as a "knowledge commons", too (Hess and Ostrom 2007, 3), where scientific know-how is embedded in and borne by the body of the animal. As such, xeno's animal commons is envisioned by involved parties as, at the very least, a temporary "collective-action initiative" (ibid., 15), sustained by, in Strathern's words, "collaborative creativity" (Strathern 2005, 19) within a research climate plagued by both a scarcity of investors and experimental failure, yet still driven by the promissory hopes and desires of porcine biocapital.

Conclusion: is there room for a human transplant commons?

I end this chapter by looping back to the theme of sharing within the domain of allotransplantation. What lessons might xeno scientists' collective actions inspire? Among the more radical turns in recent years within allotransplantation has been the rise of small collective registries of willing living donors who wish to offer a kidney to someone whom they know but where blood and tissue matching proves incompatible. Single or multiple pairs of willing donors and patients-in-need are now creating specialized networks designed to facilitate the sharing of organs among members of a donor/patient pool. For instance, if Agnes wishes to donate a kidney to her sister Ingrid, but the match is incompatible, they then join a network of four other donor/patient pairs and pool their resources. Agnes then gives her kidney to another patient, and then Ingrid gains a kidney from yet another member of the collective pool. This and still other radical forms of organ sharing are known as "paired kidney exchanges (PKEs)" and "altruistic donor chains" (Ferrari and de Klerk 2009). They define a still relatively unusual set of practices, offering evidence, I assert, of an emergent organ donor commons, one not unlike the animal commons of experimental xeno research.

If, in closing, we return once again to xeno's "what if" logic, we might begin to imagine a parallel set of possibilities for allotransplantation. What if a willingness to donate were reframed as a desire to share? What if participation in donor registries were a collaborative effort, where participants pooled medical data to generate a knowledge commons, where once personal data were now understood as shared resources? Such proposals generate an alternative means for the sharing of one's organs and, even, of oneself. Faced with the reality of chronic scarcity, the transplant industry might follow the lead of the animal commons, where donor chains – as a human commons – could well define new forms of "collaborative creativity" (again, see Strathern 2005), driven not by market principles of supply and demand, but by an open source approach to human need, sentiment and the desire to share.

Acknowledgements

I wish thank Kristin Zeiler and Erik Malmqvist for the opportunity to participate in the wonderful symposium on *Sharing Bodies within and across Borders* in beautiful Uppsala in May, 2014. They and other participants offered stimulating papers, compelling commentaries and, more generally, fun and good cheer throughout our days together. Special thanks are due, too, to the Swedish Collegium for Advanced Study, an oasis that offers a spectacular setting for academic work and respite.

Portions of the data that inform this chapter were collected with generous support from my employer, Barnard College, the Wenner-Gren Foundation for Anthropological Research (Grant no. 7010) and the National Science Foundation (any opinions, findings and conclusions or recommendations expressed in this material are mine and do not necessarily reflect the views of the National Science Foundation or other institutions).

References

Butler, D. 2002. "Xenotransplant Experts Express Caution over Knockout Piglets." *Nature* 415: 103–104.

Calne, R. 1997. "Animal Organ Transplants." *British Journal of Hospital Medicine* 57(3): 66–67.
Calne, R. 2005. "Xenografting – The Future of Transplantation, and Always Will Be?" *Xenotransplantation* 12(1): 5–6.
Cook, P.S. 2006. *Science Stories: Selecting the Source Animal for Xenotransplantation. Social Change in the 21st Century.* Queensland, Australia: Centre for Social Change Research, University of Technology.
Cooper, D.K.C., and R.P. Lanza. 2000. *Xeno: The Promise of Transplanting Animal Organs into Humans.* Oxford: Oxford University Press.
Cooper, M. 2008. *Life as Surplus: Biotechnology and Capitalism in the Neoliberal Era.* Seattle: University of Washington Press.
Corbey, R. 2005. *The Metaphysics of Apes: Negotiating the Animal–Human Boundary.* Cambridge, UK: Cambridge University Press.
d'Apice, A.J.F., Nottle, M.B., and P.J. Cowan. 2001. "Genetic Modification for Xenotransplantation: Transgenics and Clones." *Transplantation Proceedings* 33: 3053–3054.
de Burgh, J. 1998. "Saving Our Bacon: The New Animal Farm." *The Lancet* 351: 993.
Donnelley, S. 1999a. "How and Why Animals Matter." *ILAR Journal* 40(1): 22–28.
Donnelley, S. 1999b. "The Moral Landscape of Xenotransplantation (or: Casting Pearls Before Miniature, Transgenic Swine)." Paper presented at Humans and Nature Program, Cold Spring Harbor, New York, May 12.
Eagle, R. 1963. "Man Who Received Transplant of Kidney from Chimpanzee Seen in 'Good Health'." *Reading Eagle*, December 18.
Ferrari, P., and M. de Klerk. 2009. "Paired Kidney Donations to Expand the Living Donor Pool." *Journal of Nephrology* 22(6): 699–707.
First, N.L., and F.P. Haseltine. 1988. *Transgenic Animals.* Boston: Butterworth-Heinemann.
Fletcher, J.C., Robertson, J.A., and M.R. Harrison. 1986. "Primates and Anencephalics as Sources for Pediatric Organ Transplants." *Fetal Therapy* 1: 150–164.
Fox, R.C., and J.P. Swazey. 1992. *Spare Parts: Organ Replacement in American Society.* Oxford: Oxford University Press.
Franklin, S., and M. Lock. 2003. "Animation and Cessation: The Remaking of Life and Death." In: *Remaking Life and Death: Toward an Anthropology of the Biosciences*, edited by S. Franklin and M. Lock, 3–22. Santa Fe: School of American Research Press.
Guyer, J.I. 2007. "Prophecy and the Near Future: Thoughts on Macroeconomic, Evangelical, and Punctuated Time." *American Ethnologist* 34(3): 409–421.
Hacking, I. 1995. *Rewriting the Soul: Multiple Personality and the Sciences of Memory.* Princeton: Princeton University Press.
Heinemann, L.L. 2014. "For the Sake of Others: Reciprocal Webs of Obligation and the Pursuit of Transplantation as a Caring Act." *Medical Anthropology Quarterly* 28(1): 66–84.
Hess, C., and E. Ostrom. 2007. "Introduction: An Overview of the Knowledge Commons." In *Understanding Knowledge as a Commons: From Theory to Practice*, edited by C. Hess and E. Ostrom, 3–26. Cambridge, MA: MIT Press.
Hyde, L. 2010. *Common as Air: Revolution, Art, and Ownership.* New York: Farrar, Straus, and Giroux.
Jackson, M. 2002. "Familiar and Foreign Bodies: A Phenomenological Exploration of the Human–Technology Interface." *Journal of the Royal Anthropological Institute (JRAI)* 8(2): 333–346.

Kaebnick, G. 2002. "The Cloned Pigs and the 'Reality' of Xenotransplantation." *Hastings Center Report* 32(2): 7.

Kopytoff, I. 1986. "The Cultural Biography of Things: Commoditization as Process." In: *The Social Life of Things: Commodities in Cultural Perspective*, edited by A. Appadurai, 64–91. Cambridge: Cambridge University Press.

The Lancet. 1997. Editorial. "Have a Pig's Heart?" *The Lancet* 349: 219.

Lemonick, M.D. 2002. "Pig Parts for People?" *Time* 159(2): 65.

Livingston, J. 2012. *Improvising Medicine: An African Oncology Ward in an Emerging Cancer Epidemic*. Durham: Duke University Press.

Maeder, T., and P.E. Ross. 2002. "Machines for Living." *Red Herring* 113: 41–46.

Mauss, M. 1967. *The Gift: Forms and Functions of Exchange in Archaic Societies.* Translated by I. Cunnison. New York: W.W. Norton & Co., Inc.

Murray, T.H. 1987. "Gifts of the Body and the Needs of Strangers." *Hastings Center Report* 17(2): 30–38.

Nature. 1984. "Grandstand Medicine: Baboons' Hearts Are not Taboo for People, but Medicine Which Is not Essential Is Wrong." *Nature* 312 (November 8): 88.

Nelkin, D., and L. Andrews. 1998. "Homo Economicus: The Commercialization of Body Tissue in the Age of Biotechnology." *Hastings Center Report* 28(5): 30–39.

Patience, C., Takeuchi, Y., and R.A. Weiss. 1997. "Infection of Human Cells by an Endogenous Retrovirus of Pigs." *Nature Medicine* 3: 282–287.

Pollack, A. 2012. "Move to Market Gene-Altered Pigs in Canada is Halted." *New York Times*, April 4.

Richardson, R. 1996. "Fearful Symmetry: Corpses for Anatomy, Organs for Transplantation?" In: *Organ Transplantation: Meanings and Realities*, edited by R. Fox, L. O'Connell and S. Youngner, 66–100. Madison: University of Wisconsin Press.

Rose, N. 2001. "The Politics of Life Itself." *Theory, Culture and Society* 18(6): 1–30.

Rothman, D.J., Rose, E., Awaya, T., Cohen, B., Daar, A., Dzemeshkevich, S.L., Lee, C.J., Munro, R., Reyes, H., Rothman, S.M., Schoen, K.F., Scheper-Hughes, N., Shapira, Z., and H. Smit. 1997. "The Bellagio Task Force Report on Transplantation, Bodily Integrity, and the International Traffic in Organs." *Transplantation Proceedings* 29(6): 2739–2745.

Scheper-Hughes, N., and L.J.D. Wacquant, eds. 2003. *Commodifying Bodies.* Thousand Oaks, CA: Sage.

Sells, R.A. 1992. "Toward an Affordable Ethic." *Transplantation Proceedings* 24(5): 2095–2096.

Sharp, L.A. 2001. "Commodified Kin: Death, Mourning, and Competing Claims on the Bodies of Organ Donors in the United States." *American Anthropologist* 103(1): 1–21.

Sharp, L.A. 2002. "Denying Culture in the Transplant Arena: Technocratic Medicine's Myth of Democratization." *Cambridge Quarterly of Healthcare Ethics* 11(2): 142–150.

Sharp, L.A. 2006a. "Babes and Baboons: Jesica Santillan and Experimental Pediatric Transplant Research in America." In: *Beyond the Bungled Transplant – Jesica Santillan and High Tech Medicine in Cultural Perspective*, edited by K. Wailoo, P. Guarnaccia and J. Livingston, 299–328. Chapel Hill: The University of North Carolina Press.

Sharp, L.A. 2006b. *Strange Harvest: Organ Transplants, Denatured Bodies, and the Transformed Self.* Berkeley: University of California Press.

Sharp, L.A. 2007. *Bodies, Commodities, and Biotechnologies: Death, Mourning, and Scientific Desire in the Realm of Human Organ Transfer.* New York: Columbia University Press.

Sharp, L.A. 2013. *The Transplant Imaginary: Mechanical Hearts, Animal Parts, and Moral Thinking in Highly Experimental Science.* Berkeley: University of California Press.

Sharp, L.A. 2014. "Perils Before Swine: Biosecurity and Scientific Longing in Experimental Xenotransplant Research." In: *Bioinsecurity and Vulnerability*, edited by N. Chen and L.A. Sharp, 45–64. Santa Fe: SAR Press.

Siminoff, L.A., and K. Chillag. 1999. "The Fallacy of the 'Gift of Life'." *Hastings Center Report* 29(6): 34–41.

Starzl, T.E., and J. Fung. 1993. "Baboon-to-Human Liver Transplantation." *The Lancet* 341(8837): 65–71.

Strathern, M. 2005. "Imagined Collectivities and Multiple Authorship." In: *CODE: Collaborative Ownership and the Digital Economy*, edited by R.A. Ghosh, 13–28. Cambridge MA: MIT Press.

Sunder Rajan, K. 2006. *Biocapital: The Constitution of Postgenomic Life.* Durham: Duke University Press.

Sunder Rajan, K. 2012. *Lively Capital: Biotechnologies, Ethics, and Governance in Global Markets.* Durham: Duke University Press.

Sypniewski, D., Machnik, G., Mazurek, U., Wilczok, T., Smorag, Z., Jura, J., and B. Gajda. 2005. "Distribution of Porcine Endogenous Retroviruses (PERVs) DNA in Organs of Domestic Pig." *Annals of Transplantation* 10(2): 46–51.

Thompson, E.P. 1993. *Customs in Common: Studies in Traditional Popular Culture.* New York: The New Press.

Waldby, C., and R. Mitchell. 2006. *Tissue Economies: Blood, Organs, and Cell Lines in Late Capitalism.* Durham: Duke University Press.

Weiss, R.A. 1998. "Retroviral Zoonoses." *Nature Medicine* 4: 391–392.

Wendland, C. 2010. *A Heart for the Work: Journeys through an African Medical School.* Chicago: University of Chicago Press.

7 Sharing the embodied experience of pregnancy

The case of surrogate motherhood

Sarah Jane Toledano

Introduction

> The baby moves. My hand goes to my rounded belly, my entire hand, palm down, pressing lightly. There is the cloth of my clothing beneath my hand, but my hand doesn't feel it. There is the skin of my abdomen beneath the cloth, but my hand doesn't feel it. I touch the cloth and the skin beneath it, but what I feel is the baby. I take the hands of my husband or my sister, but I don't say: "Here, feel my dress move, or feel my belly move." Rather, I say: "Feel the baby." I gently place their hands on my abdomen, palms rounded, flat, as much of their palms to my tummy as possible, skin to skin, so they have a better chance of feeling what I feel from the inside.
>
> (Van der Zalm 2011)

In her classic essay, "Pregnant Embodiment: Subjectivity and Alienation", Iris Marion Young (1984, 45) claimed that "discourse on pregnancy omits subjectivity, for the specific experience of women has been absent from most of our culture's discourse about human experience". However, this claim is hardly true anymore. Scholarship on pregnant embodiment has shown remarkable progress in recent years, and the experience of childbearing has come to be recognized as a fruitful source of insight to theorize on social and ethical relations (Baraitser 2009; Mullin 2005). An increasing number of female scholars have included subjective accounts of pregnant embodiment in their theoretical work (Bigwood 1991; Lintott and Sander-Staudt 2012; Tyler 2000).

In spite of this scholarly progress, much is left to be explored about pregnancy in terms of how the changing technological landscape in which we find ourselves could create variances of pregnant embodiment – of the bodies that could be pregnant, for whom one can be pregnant and with whom a pregnancy is meaningfully experienced – that complicate previous conceptualizations, challenge normative understandings and expand on the diversity of the lived experience of pregnancy. For example, technologies that assist reproduction, practices that allow for the adoption of another's frozen embryos, surrogate motherhood and the recent success of uterus transplantation illustrate the potential relations that are enabled and the customarily relied-on norms that are contested when these practices expand the domain of those who could be invested in a pregnancy. Such technologies, for example, recall assumptions implicitly found in theoretical works on pregnant embodiment: that the pregnant subject is generally presumed to be the one who will also rear the child upon birth, or that the relationship in pregnancy centrally revolves around the maternal–foetal relation.

In this chapter, I explore a potential variance in pregnant embodiment through the case of gestational surrogate pregnancies, as a way of reframing the focus on pregnant embodiment from one that is centred on the maternal–foetal dyadic relation into one that more pronouncedly illustrates the other relational multiplicities that are meaningfully created during pregnancy. By making certain relational multiplicities more nuanced, I also seek to draw attention to how sharing occurs in pregnancy; specifically, how others are able to empathize, or to feel-with another's subjective experience. I take it that, while assisted reproductive technologies (ARTs) and surrogate motherhood have been problematic within feminist ethics, they also provide a venue for navigating through different emerging understandings of maternal bodies, maternal experiences and social relations, because of the non-conventional route in which families are created through them. As such, they also hold the promise of challenging generalized characterizations of reproductive experiences. My theoretical starting point is a revisiting of Iris Marion Young's characterization of pregnant embodiment, from which I advance the view that the intersubjective space of sharing in pregnant embodiment expands beyond the embodied relationship between the pregnant subject and the foetus.

Revisiting Young: pregnant embodiment as a privileged relation

Many of the existing works that deal with pregnant embodiment ground their discussion on the formative phenomenological characterization of gendered pregnant embodiment developed by Iris Marion Young (1984; 2005). The ubiquity of Young's characterization to the field of philosophical and empirical research of pregnancy cannot be ignored. Young's essay is part of her larger work of illuminating distinctive female bodily experiences in order to challenge gender-neutral phenomenological descriptions and dichotomizing conceptions of the self, such as the subject–object mode of bodily being. The *subject–object mode of bodily being* refers to the alienated objectification that the subject experiences whenever the body is brought to an awareness of its "weight and materiality" – the body becoming *other*, an impediment to one's projects, and an object in the external world rather than the subject that enacts the world (Young 1984, 50). Young contends that pregnancy draws the subject to her physicality through the bodily changes and sensations, but that these could nevertheless be experienced positively.[1] By bringing to light the specific lived bodily experience of what she identifies as "chosen pregnancies in technologically sophisticated Western societies", Young characterizes pregnancy as a *splitting subjectivity*:

> The pregnant subject is decentered, split or doubled in several ways, experiences her body as herself and not herself. Its inner movements belong to another being, yet they are not other, because her body boundaries shift and because her bodily self-location is focused on her trunk in addition to her head.
>
> (ibid., 46)

Young claims that the movements of the foetus and the pregnant subject's changing body shape and mass condition her experience and spatial orientation, and undermine her bodily integrity (ibid., 48). All these effects are experienced by the pregnant subject alone, who is described to have the "privileged relation to this other life, not unlike that I have to my dreams and thoughts, which I can tell someone, but which cannot be an object for both of us in some way" (ibid., 48). Her growing body during pregnancy is the only immediately visible sign to others of the dynamic, dialectical process occurring within her (ibid., 54).

This unique mode of experience that no one else can share is reiterated by Young in a postscript to her work written in 2003. In spite of the significant technological changes of the time, this particular character of pregnant embodiment has not changed:

> she *is* a pregnant person; it is she and only she who lives this growing body and moves within it. She and only she has a privileged relation of *feeling* with the developing fetus. The pregnant woman feels the weight, position, and motion of the fetus as part of herself yet not herself. Others have access to feeling this developing life only by contact with and through her.
>
> (Young 2005, 61; emphasis in original)[2]

Upholding this privileged embodied relationship could be understood based on how Young sought to bring to the fore the subjective experiences of women, and on her critique of the practices and technologies in obstetrical and gynaecological medicine that had devalued women's own accounts of their pregnant experience (Young 1984, 45). The pregnant subject's own reports of her feelings and descriptions of her felt sensations of the foetus were seen at that time to have been replaced by medical technologies such as foetal imaging, which were taken by the obstetrical and gynaecological profession to have a more substantive and credible epistemological role. This alienating attitude by the obstetrical field toward the subjective experience of women is explained by Young as partly owing to the notion that "pregnancy and childbirth entail a unique body subjectivity which is difficult to empathize with unless one is or has been pregnant" (Young 1984, 58).

Beyond the maternal–foetal relation in pregnant embodiment

Young's phenomenological characterization has been treated as canonical, and very few who engaged in exploring the embodied experience of pregnancy have questioned her phenomenological characterization of chosen pregnancies (Oliver 2010; Lundquist 2008). However, she admits that her account of female body experience is in no way definitive (Young 2005). It is in this openness to potential gaps that significant directions to extend inquiries of pregnant embodiment beyond her framing of positively experienced maternal–foetal relations in chosen pregnancies become fruitful. After all, one can speculate on the complex ways by which pregnancies are lived by pregnant subjects – even those that can be said to be chosen pregnancies – and the situation that makes them experience their pregnancies in a particular way. This is, for example, the analytic work that is offered by Caroline Lundquist (2008) who advanced an account of unwanted, rejected and denied pregnancies. She illustrates the phenomenological experience of "being torn" among pregnant subjects in unwanted and rejected pregnancies rather than that of a positive identification and splitting subjectivity (ibid., 140). She explains that pregnant subjects who have unwanted pregnancies have an objectifying, alienating regard toward the foetus – it is seen as an "annoyance", an "intrusion", or "some unwanted or menacing object, some less than human, perhaps monstrous creature or the embodiment of the aggressor, in pregnancies resulting from rape" (ibid., 41). In spite of the difference in context from Young's chosen pregnancies, what Lundquist seeks to bring out in her work is the recognition of phenomenological discourses in pregnancy as "tentative descriptive categories" even as they tend toward describing modes of experience (ibid., 137). This recognition provides leeway to problematize and supplement Young's account, allowing for more expansive theoretical discourses on pregnant embodiment.

Another author who engages with and questions Young's characterization of splitting subjectivity is Gail Weiss, who discusses, based on her own pregnant experience, how pregnancy need not necessarily undermine bodily integrity, and how it actually *resignifies* our perspective of the boundaries of the self – the body can be understood as fluid and expansive through the very changes that it undergoes in life, rather than as a whole and enclosed body in which changes appear to be transgressions to bodily integrity (Weiss 1999, 53). Talia Welsh (2008) is supportive of Weiss's (1999) view on bodily integrity, and also of Carol Bigwood's (1991) conceptualization of the body as a presence that weaves itself into other relations in the world. The insights of both these scholars are inspired by their own pregnant experiences. In particular, Welsh's (2008) idea of a self that is essentially and inextricably connected to others and the world, rather than existing as a self-enclosed and bounded being, could be a promising direction for understanding the interplay of our own bodily experiences within a larger social world.

I take these works that engage and question Young's work seriously, in so far as they open further investigations of the diversity of pregnant embodiment and re-emphasize the intersubjective (relational) conception of the self found in phenomenological scholarship. They also challenge the degree of privacy and solitariness by which women experience their pregnancies. This is not to say that relationality does not figure in Young's account; however, Young's descriptions of the embodied relationship shared by the pregnant subject and the foetus tend to define pregnancy as a centrally and meaningfully dyadic relationship. According to Young's viewpoint, others – particularly those who have not had a prior experience of pregnancy – could find it quite challenging to become part of this dyadic relationship.

I think that if one limited one's understanding of empathy to situations where one has had an exactly similar first-person experience, then it would truly be difficult to accept that others who have not gone through a similar bodily experience could still feel deeply and intensely along with the person having the experience. Such an understanding of empathy would also narrow the extent to which significant relations forged during pregnancy were able to meaningfully affect a pregnant experience. Yet as shown in the work of Lundquist (2008), other relations are able to shape the lived bodily experience of the pregnant subject, and affect the meanings that she grants to the developing foetus. It does not necessarily follow that being able to affect somebody per se means that one is actively sharing that person's experience. However, the ability of others to affect a pregnant experience draws attention to a conception of the self in pregnancy that involves being part of a "larger sense of life that exceeds a single body" (Welsh 2008, 54), and that concretizes the possibility of the participation of others into one's lived experience.

Sharing another's embodied experience

I engage with the notion of the lived body that has become a base of Young's work on gendered embodiment in order to explore the different ways in which pregnancy is experienced by women in their specific subjective situations and within their self-enacted projects. This engagement with the lived body also serves the analytic purpose of clarifying the ways in which our relations with others are intertwined, which in turn allows for scrutiny of the creation (or even transgression) of a sharing context during pregnancy.

The non-dualistic conception of the self, as propounded by the phenomenology of Maurice Merleau-Ponty (1962), underscores our engagement with the world as embodied selves or lived bodies. Our perception of the world and our orientation within it are due to our embodiment – the unification of our mind and body. We are intertwined with a world that is shared and co-constituted with others, and which we relate to through concrete lived situations rather than by experiencing them as cognitive and purely separate facets of human existence. As constituting subjects and not pure objects of the world (Csordas 1990), we are engaged in constant meaning-making, in an intersubjective relation with fellow embodied selves.

Those working within the perspective of the phenomenology of the body have already explored the idea that the inherently relational character of human existence causes our engagement with the world to involve a basic giving to and receiving from each other in ways that are not always thematically or consciously present to us – yet through which we become attuned to each other, incorporate skills and develop habits (see Zeiler 2014a, 2014b). In this sense, there is a pre-reflective engagement with the given world in which we are already fundamentally involved in "sharing our bodily existence in different ways", that is, a mode of giving-through-sharing that takes place despite the asymmetries of our embodied selves (Zeiler 2014b, 178). However, our intersubjective relationships with others as fellow lived bodies maintain our singular selves, rather than causing them to be dissolved (Käll forthcoming; van Hooft 2003). The notion of sharing another's embodied experience is not impossible when one considers that we are already participating, both pre-reflectively and reflectively, in each other's meaning-making and ways of being in the world.[3]

We understand each other through the visible expressions of our experiences, such as bodily behaviour and gestures; and these expressions transpire within concrete situations and meaningful contexts (Zahavi 2001). Our daily lives show that "we understand each other well enough through our shared engagement in the common world" without any rigorous effort to do so (Zahavi 2001, 155). While one's understanding of another person's experience is incommensurable to the first-person lived experience, this difference or asymmetry does not deny one's "ability to access the life of the mind of others in their expressive behavior and meaningful action" (Zahavi 2011, 10). This very difference or asymmetry of our embodied selves also preserves the phenomenological stance that we encounter others in their *alterity* or radical otherness – that is, we confront another who is also an embodied self, but who is different from us and who cannot be appropriated or projected onto as a person wholly similar to ourselves (Levinas 1969; Zahavi 2001).

Thus, first-hand subjective experiences that are presented as being singular, private and solitary to the individual are not necessarily exempted from being touched by the participation of others in a way that can affect the bodily experience. We resonate to the embarrassment, shame, pain, joys and pleasures of others because we have had such emotions ourselves in different concrete situations, and are thus able to recognize them in the experiences of others in their own specific situations. The shared experience of being embodied subjects allows us to respond to and commiserate with other people out of empathy, understood as "feeling-with" them (see Kruks 2001). To *feel-with* others is to have an affective response toward their experience, without presupposing and appropriating that one is actually feeling what the other is feeling (ibid.). Feeling-with another's experiential situation is an intersubjective encounter that preserves the subjectivity of persons and respects the first-person lived experience. It is motivated by perceptible and communicable expressions of the others' subjectivity, because lived experiences are visibly and communicably expressed. For example, pain is regarded as private and both ineffable to and ungraspable by others. Scholars suggest that the responses of others toward the one suffering from pain – how others feel-with the suffering other – significantly affect how the pain becomes magnified or eased for this person (Scarry 1985; Käll 2013).

The experience of pregnancy is similar to this view on pain. Pregnancy has been identified as a private experience of the pregnant subject (Trobe 2013; Michaels 1996). She is the one who is able to feel the sensations of the developing foetus directly, and to experience the travails of carrying the gestating child to term and the pains of labour. While all these bodily experiences are the pregnant subject's alone, the visibility of her form communicates to others the heaviness of the pregnancy and can even solicit a response. If she so desires, she can create a shared space where others can access the growing life within her through touch (Young 2005, 61). Without any reflective thought or discussion between parties, situations exist where those who have not experienced pregnancy or birthing pains have still been observed to feel-with the woman in labour and to "reciprocally push" with her during the birth process (see LaChance Adams and Burcher 2014).

The notions of the lived body and of empathy respect Young's noble aim of advancing women's authority through their personal knowledge of their pregnancy, while allowing for a shared space in which others become participants and not just spectators during pregnancy. Certain problematic implications of her work – such as the idea that males, who have not and cannot be pregnant, cannot share the lived experience of pregnant subjects; or that a pregnant experience needs to be mediated by the pregnant subject in order to be understood or felt-with by others – are addressed by the understanding that empathy, as "feeling-with" another does not deny the incomparable first-person experience, but is rather the affective response of others to the pregnant subject in her own situation. A tendency to set the commonality of childbearing capacity and experience as necessary conditions for empathy comparably diminishes the depth of the felt attachment that others can have to the pregnant subject and the developing child-to-be; it also under-appreciates the care and concern that significant others can have toward the pregnancy.

Exploring empathy in terms of feeling-with another's lived experience could illustrate the sharing that takes place during pregnancy and that expands pregnant embodiment beyond the dyadic privileged relation of the pregnant subject with the gestating child. Thus, being able to feel-with another's lived experience of pregnancy becomes less dependent on shared fixtures of a body and more dependent on the interpersonal gestures by which others become attuned to the behaviour, needs and vulnerabilities of pregnant subjects. Moreover, going beyond understanding pregnancy as an exclusive and privileged relation also avoids any potential overgeneralization of a chosen pregnancy as a positive bodily experience that is always "noticed and savored for its own sake" (Young 1984, 47). Such claims could adversely impact pregnant subjects by reinforcing the intuitive expectation that they are able to form a deep-seated attachment with the developing foetus due to their privileged corporeal relation, and that they *should* then form a bond and attachment with the child.

Carrying a child for another

With these above-mentioned considerations, I would like to reflect on the case of gestational surrogate pregnancy in order to contribute to a variant of pregnant embodiment and to make an analysis of the thoughtful work of sharing the subjective experience of pregnancy. Gestational surrogate motherhood is a practice made possible by advances in assisted reproductive technologies, in which an individual – the surrogate mother – agrees to become pregnant through in vitro fertilization (IVF) upon a prior agreement that the parental rights to the resulting child will be transferred to the intended parents (Brazier *et al.*, 1998). In this type of surrogacy, there is no genetic connection between the resulting child and the surrogate mother. The gametes used in IVF typically come from the intended parents themselves or are donor gametes. Depending on the legislation of the state or country, the intended parents in surrogate motherhood are typically heterosexual and same-sex couples where one (as in the female) or both (as in gay men) cannot carry a pregnancy due to a malfunctional or absent uterus, recurrent miscarriages, numerous failed IVF implantations, or health dangers in childbearing.

In the context of surrogate motherhood, where there is a prior agreement that the pregnant subject is not to be the child-rearer, what would be the character of the embodied relationship between the pregnant subject and the developing foetus? How can we understand the meaning of experiencing a "privileged relation with the fetus and her pregnant body" (Young 1984, 46)? If the embodied maternal–foetal relationship is an experience that "no one can share" unless mediated by the pregnant subject, what does it entail for the pregnant subject to engage others, specifically the intended parents, in her pregnant experience (Young 2005, 61)? What are the implications to her subjectivity – to her way of being-in-the-world? While there is strong opposition from some feminists to surrogate motherhood (see Raymonds 1993; Narayan 1995), I align myself to the view of Meredith Michaels: that there can be an analysis of the transformative potential of reproductive technologies that is at "odds with, but remains appreciative of, the character of these feminist debates" (Michaels 1996, 50).

The various procedures and processes that are required in order to engage in surrogate motherhood already disrupt traditional understandings of reproduction as belonging in the private arena of the couple. They also pluralize categories of parenthood, and challenge the taken-for-granted expectation that mothers who choose to gestate a child will also be the child-rearers. Considering these relational complexities in surrogacy, I first turn to two data points found in previous empirical studies of the lived experience of gestational surrogate mothers, in order to examine the mode of sharing that takes place in their pregnant embodiment. I then elaborate on the mode of sharing that occurs within them.

The first data point occurs in the context of commercial surrogate arrangements in Israel, as discussed by Elly Teman (2009). Teman describes the mutual collaborative identity work between the surrogate mother and the intended mother. In Israel, financial payments and state mediation are involved in surrogate arrangements. The surrogates and intended mothers in this particular study engaged in a *dyadic body project*, in which the intended mother actively engaged in embodying the surrogate's pregnancy, while the surrogate actively transferred her pregnant experience to the intended mother and distanced herself from any maternal identity (Teman 2009, 50). The experience of the pregnancy, in terms of the foetal movements and sensations, was communicated and transferred to the intended mother for her to embody it as her own. Teman labelled this conscious process of detaching and disembodying as the *shifting body* (ibid., 49). Through this shifting body, the joint body project involved essential activities that the surrogates and the intended mothers shared together so that both of them could embody the respective identity they wanted for themselves (ibid., 65). Teman also described the expected "shared 'holding'" of the pregnancy between these women (ibid., 62). Shared holding occurred when intended mothers reciprocally responded and positively accepted the ways that the surrogates channelled the pregnancy to them. This holding on the part of the intended mother was believed to have implications for the progress of the surrogate pregnancy. As explained by one surrogate mother who miscarried in the study, the miscarriage was because the intended mother "didn't help me hold it! And it fell!" (ibid., 62). This transpired in a case where an intended mother secretly and successfully had herself implanted with her remaining embryos and did not feel the need to bond with the surrogate anymore.

The shifting body and the expected shared holding were the means by which the surrogates differentiated their pre-pregnant self-identity from their temporary role as a gestational carrier; these activities also actively engaged the intended mother to bond with her child. From the perspective of the intended mothers, the wombs of the surrogates were extensions of their bodies, like a "prosthetic consciousness"; this situation was made analogous to Merleau-Ponty's depiction of a walking stick as an extension of a blind person's body (Teman 2010, 140).[4] Teman characterized this as a "relationship of encompassment", where the intended mother perceives the body of the surrogate as servicing her project of being a mother to her biological child (ibid., 168).

At this point, I cite the case of Ayala and Sima as a data point in Teman's (2009) study. Ayala, the intended mother for Sima's surrogacy, described her experience of the pregnant embodiment of Sima as follows:

> What she goes through, I also go through … And we speak a lot about these things, *and she is a partner in this, we are together, we are one body together* now, that is what I want to say. We are one body together that is pregnant with twins.
>
> (Teman 2009, 60; emphasis in original)

Sima, the surrogate, had an initial appreciation of Ayala's involvement, and took this as an empathizing and nurturing stance toward her situation.

However, Sima was ultimately described to have felt the intense surveillance, overprotectiveness and proximity of the intended parents as suffocating; she felt like an "object" and a "prisoner in their home and prisoner within her own body" (ibid., 61).

The other data point occurs in the context of altruistic surrogate motherhood arrangements between families and friends. No payment is involved in this kind of surrogate arrangement. It has been claimed that there is a paucity of data looking into "how the actors involved in surrogacy experience, understand, and verbalize these relationships" and this is undeniably the case for altruistic surrogacy between close interpersonal relations such as families and friends (Pande 2009, 381).

Elsewhere, a colleague and I focus on this specific form of surrogate arrangement, and discuss the reciprocal relational work between the surrogate mothers and the intended parents (Toledano and Zeiler forthcoming). The surrogate mothers who were interviewed for that study described the sense of embodied responsibility that they felt during the surrogate pregnancy. They also emphasized the surrogacy as an other-regarding gesture, which they offered for the sake of their friend or relative whose struggles in having a child were witnessed by them. The relational work of the surrogate mothers was also understood from how they described the *boundary-setting efforts* of disconnecting the pregnancy from their husbands and sharing the pregnant experience with the intended parents, particularly with the intended mother. They made these efforts by encouraging the intended parents to touch their pregnant bellies and by updating them on the sensations from their developing foetus. This activity was also performed in order to have the parents embody touching *their* child. The bonding and emotions that the surrogate mothers reported to have felt toward the child-to-be were described as being a different experience from that of their own pregnancies with their own children.

From this study, I cite the data point of Ashley, who was a surrogate mother for her cousin. Ashley stated that she did not exactly know what it was like to be in the position of her cousin, who had gone through numerous failed IVF treatments, and that she offered the surrogacy in light of what she described as a "privileged position" to have had uncomplicated pregnancies and through which she saw herself as being able to help the intended parents. Her surrogate pregnancy ended in miscarriage; and even though she had been pregnant before, and the surrogate pregnancy was an other-regarding gesture toward the intended parents, she described how the miscarriage deeply affected her. She had cared for the surrogate pregnancy in more ways than she did when she gestated her own children, and was very affected by the devastating impact the miscarriage would have on the intended parents.

These two different contexts of surrogacy and these two specific data points are taken as concrete situations within the broad practice of surrogate motherhood, and add to the variances of pregnant embodiment. Gestational surrogate pregnancies illustrate how the giving of self is realized through the intersubjective encounter between the pregnant subject and the intended parents. The surrogacy enters them into a relation with each other in which the pregnant embodiment is highly significant for the stakeholders. The surrogate experience strongly illustrates how the intersubjective relations in pregnancy include the maternal–foetal dyad of the pregnant subject and the gestating child without excluding the roles of other constituting relations. These significant relations can be seen to shape the pregnant subject's lived experience of the surrogate pregnancy, and challenge understandings of pregnant embodiment as "interior" or "privately suffered" (Michaels 1996, 62).[5] In both of the cases described above, sharing the pregnancy with one or both of the intended parents involved an openness to each other that was made evident in how the surrogate mothers allowed the touching of their bellies as a way for the intended parents to feel-with them and with their child. Allowing their bellies to be touched can also be understood to describe how the surrogate mothers felt-with any potential fears of the intended parents, as well as the surrogate mothers' need to assuage the parents' concerns that the surrogates might develop threatening maternal attachments that could affect the future relinquishment of the child. The affective dimension of sharing the subjectivity of the other is emphasized in the initiating move of the surrogate mothers to have the intended parents bond with and feel with them the sensations of their gestating child. It is an intertwining of their intersubjective selves in lieu of their bodily asymmetries – their respective subjectivities – to feel together the gestating foetus. Pregnant embodiment in this sense no longer strictly takes place in Young's sense of a privileged relation that the pregnant subject has with the developing child and her pregnant body, especially when the meaning of the pregnancy is strongly presented to be an other-regarding gesture toward others who are emotionally invested in it (Young 1984, 46).

In spite of the intended mothers and the surrogate mothers appearing in foreign situations to each other, because the former either have not had an experience of pregnancy or have lost or lacked childbearing abilities, while the latter have experienced at least one successful pregnancy, their unique embodiment and asymmetries make possible their work of sharing the pregnancy by feeling-with each other's situation. The first case portrays the creative body interaction between surrogates and intended mothers as they co-inhabit an imagined shared space in which they shift bodies to co-create their self-chosen maternal identities. The disembodying disposition of the surrogate mothers toward the pregnancy is the embodying path given to the intended mother, granting security and assurance of a maternal identity. *They* – Ayala and Sima – are pregnant, and one goes through what the other goes through in the process. The second case, that of the altruistic surrogacy, highlights the surrogate mother's feeling-with her friend or relative's struggles and hopes to have a child. Instead of taking her "privileged position" of having successfully born a child as distinctively and exclusively hers, Ashley took it in relation to her cousin's differential situation. She felt-with her cousins' situation by recognizing and acknowledging that although she had never been in their situation of being unable to bear a child, she could nevertheless help them through her own bodily capacity. The gravity of the miscarriage was regarded by her not as a felt loss of a precious personal possession, for which she could grieve, but rather as the loss and grief of the intended parents.

However, from within this shared space of pregnant embodiment, where it has been expectedly the case that there will be a reciprocal and conducive surrogacy context for one another, the asymmetries in embodiment also have the potential to lead to the transgression of the other's subjectivity. It has been pointed out earlier that feeling-with another's embodied subjectivity as a mode of sharing does not necessitate a perfect or guaranteed similarity of experience. A need for a "respectful recognition" has been suggested in light of being singular selves within a shared human existence (Kruks 2001, 154). The case of Ayala and Sima illustrated that a positive sharing context of feeling-with another's situation could not be a one-time event, but would require continuous work; otherwise, it would lead to an appropriation of the other's subjectivity and projection of the self's vested interest. Ayala, in her self-project of thoroughly encompassing motherhood, transformed from being perceived as a nurturer and reciprocal partner in the dyadic body project into a subject that objectified the surrogate mother and transgressed her subjectivity. It was only in the surrogate mother's distinct embodiment that Ayala could create her vision of being a mother to her biological child, and instead of a cooperative shared holding of the pregnancy (a "we"), there occurred a strong sense of ownership toward the surrogate – a "colonialization" of Sima's body and life (Teman 2009, 61).

Furthermore and along related lines, if sharing as feeling-with the other can be understood from both the altruistic and commercial surrogacy cases as being responsive to what the other lacks or needs, there is an implied dependency relation. This raises questions about who gives more in surrogacy, and what the expectations are in the differential giving to and receiving from one another in surrogacy. Here, one could consider the case of miscarriages in surrogacy. One can only speculate on the occurrence of self-blame on the part of the surrogate mothers, in which they try to account for what they could have done to prevent the miscarriage; there was also that instance of miscarriage in Teman's study, when the intended mother was blamed for not holding the pregnancy reciprocally. Additionally, without trivializing in any way the travails of the intended parents in their quest to have a child, the surrogate mothers are the ones who carry the child, as well as any unintended or intended pressures that the surrogacy will not be another dashed hope for the intended parents. As found in the case of Ashley, feeling-with the intended parents' struggles initiated the offer of the surrogacy, and also understandably created the experience of feeling-with their loss, in spite of the fact that both the pregnancy and the miscarriage were physically undergone and felt by *her* body.

It is also worth mentioning that although both the contexts of paid and unpaid surrogate arrangements evoke the beauty and asymmetries of sharing between persons, their respective contexts raise varying notions of how stakeholders partake in the sharing of pregnancy. One wonders if the involvement of payment implies a greater tendency to objectify and appropriate the pregnant subject, in the sense of being able to dispense with a perceived paid service, such as in the case of the failed shared holding in Teman's study. On the other hand, one could also wonder how the non-involvement of compensation and profit, coupled with having a surrogacy for a close personal relation, imply a greater burden of managing the surrogacy within the intuitive understanding that family relations are social settings in which one does not expect to be paid, and where one expects a certain attunement to one another's needs.

Despite these differences, it is still promising to see both surrogate situations through the lens of sharing, in which both distinctly illustrate different ways of giving and receiving within the shared goal of creating a child for another's sake. Both portray a state of feeling-with another, and the affective response that goes with this empathy involves thoughtful work and respectful recognition. In both cases, a failure in thoughtfulness and respect also show an infringement of the other's subjectivity. These two cases also illustrate how, rather than characterizing pregnant embodiment as either a positive or a negative bodily experience, it can perhaps best be characterized as a complex, layered experience with others that redraws the sense of the fluidity or even boundaries of the pregnant subject.

Conclusion

In this chapter, I have drawn attention to how the subjective experience of pregnancy can be shared by others in such a way that pregnancy is not necessarily a privileged relation of the pregnant subject. I took an approach that considered a more expansive notion of the self, based on the phenomenological understanding of embodiment being intersubjectively situated with others and with the world. In this viewpoint, sharing is already basic to coexistence. This framework, resting on phenomenological insights, recognizes that the singularity of lives is not a hindrance to understanding and sharing with one another's respective subjectivities. This framework is also important for addressing Young's issue of how bodily experiences are alienating to others, by reconsidering the different ways through which others are able to feel-with and understand the lived experience of pregnant subjects. Through Young's own point that a pregnant subject could engage in embodied expressions of her subjective lived experience, and through others' attunement to one's situation, sharing the subjective lived experience of pregnancy is possible. As such, pregnant embodiment can be seen as an ethically significant encounter with others beyond the work of birthing a child, and need not be a solitary experience that is born by the pregnant subject alone. In the specific case of gestational surrogate motherhood, I underscored how pregnancy is a shared and shareable experience between surrogate mothers and the intended mothers/parents, through their concrete interpersonal acts of engaging with each other. In the more general case of pregnant embodiment, I also put forth a variance of pregnant embodiment that has been instigated by technological advances that disrupt traditional normative understandings of self–other relations in pregnancy. The ARTs that allow for the reality of surrogacy complicate Young's conceptualization of positively identified chosen pregnancies, by creating relational complexities beyond the maternal–foetal dyad, and by challenging the taken-for-granted character of these relations. For example, surrogacy illustrates that women can consciously choose pregnancies for the sake of previously unknown persons, or in order to help bring a child into the world that is not to be a part of the pregnant subject's own nuclear family. Surrogate motherhood also illustrates how the core relation in pregnant embodiment is not focally and crucially around the maternal–foetal dyad, but can be more about the dyadic relation between the surrogate and intended mother, as in Teman's study, or pluralized even further to include both the intended parents, as exemplified in the unpaid surrogacy case. These cases also present different forms of attachment embodied during pregnancy.

Inasmuch as feeling-with another's embodied subjectivity can be taken in the positive direction of being sensitive to the ways in which our conduct affects others, I also argue for a critical interrogation on the problematic aspects of sharing, and specifically on the fragility of giving in situations where transgressions or disrespect toward another's subjectivity can equally take place from those very asymmetries and dependencies that make feeling-with another possible. Informed by the data points in this chapter, I point toward reflections on how sharing is imbedded with disproportionate giving and the burdens that come with giving one's (or a part of one's) self to others. It is also worthwhile to consider how regulations that oversee relations between people (i.e. contractual agreements, surrogacy procedures and screening) have implications for the extent of control and authority that others can wield toward the pregnant subject, and for how the generosity of specific lived bodies can potentially be exploited by others who stand to gain from them.

Acknowledgements

I would like to thank the local and international members of the research project, "Toward an Ethics of Bodily Giving and Sharing in Medicine" for their helpful comments on this work.

Notes

1 Zeiler (2010), in her phenomenological analysis of bodily self-awareness, identifies this positive, non-alienating experience as an *eu-appearance,* in contrast to Drew Leder's (1990) terms of bodily dis-appearance and dys-appearance. The former refers to a pre-reflective awareness of the body, while the latter speaks of the mode of attending to the body in occasions of discomfort and illness.

2 It is notable that Young's postscript to her essay, dated 2003, does not mention how the emergent assisted reproductive technologies and their complex procedures that

had been ethically controversial during the 1980s could have profound effects on pregnant experience or intensify aspects of her own phenomenological characterization.

3 Some of these phenomenological insights have been used as analytic tools in recent studies that engage with inquiries relating to shared embodiment. Examples include the implications of direct intercorporeal exchanges in biomedicine via tissue transfer (Waldby 2002), a father's attempt to draw a corporeal connection with his child during gestation (Boström 2012), the relational dynamics during intense face-to-face intercorporeality that draws differently abled bodies to have meaningful joint activity in dementia care (Zeiler 2014b), and how one is able to act compassionately to suffering others (Draper *et al.* 2014).

4 I thank Kristin Zeiler for pointing out that Teman's interpretation of this aspect of Merleau-Ponty's phenomenology does not strictly follow from Merleau-Ponty's discussion that the walking stick is supposed to recede from reflective awareness and be experienced eventually as a taken-for-granted (a pre-reflective) part of the man's body.

5 Amy Mullin (2005) noted that a woman's experience of pregnancy is said to depend on several factors, such as her motivations for being pregnant, her socio-economic resources, the extent of the choice to have the pregnancy and to continue it, the degree and depth of the physical changes, her attitude to her pre-pregnant body image and the response of significant others and the community.

References

Baraitser, L. 2009. *Maternal Encounters: The Ethics of Interruption.* London and New York: Routledge.

Bigwood, C. 1991. "Renaturalizing the Body (with the Help of Merleau-Ponty)." *Hypatia* 6(3): 54–73.

Boström, E.J. 2012. "Intersubjectivity – How to Create the Other From the Second." Paper presented at the conference Phenomenology of Pregnancy and Drives – Erotic Intersubjectivity. Södertörn University, Stockholm, April 18–20.

Brazier, M., Campbell, A., and S. Golombok. 1998. Surrogacy: Review for Health Ministers of Current Arrangements for Payments and Regulation. Report of the Review Team. Available at: http://webarchive.nationalarchives.gov.uk/+/www.dh.gov.uk/en/Publicationsandstatistics/Publications/PublicationsLegislation/DH_4009697.

Csordas, T. 1990. "Embodiment as a Paradigm for Anthropology." *Ethos* 18(1): 5–47.

Draper, M., Polizzi, D., Breton, B., Glenn, K., and J. Ogilvie. 2014. "Shared Embodiment and Shared Conversation: Compassion in Clinical Forensics." *Journal of Theoretical and Philosophical Criminology* 6(1): 77–101.

Käll, L. 2013. "Intercorporeality and the Sharability of Pain." In: *Dimensions of Pain*, edited by Lisa Käll, 27–40. London and New York: Routledge.

Käll, L. Forthcoming. "Intercorporeal Expression and the Subjectivity of Dementia." In: *Body/Self/Other: The Phenomenology of Social Encounters*, edited by L. Dolezal and D. Petherbridge. Albany, NY: SUNY Press.

Kruks, S. 2001. *Retrieving Experience. Subjectivity and Recognition in Feminist Politics.* Ithaca, NY: Cornell University Press.

LaChance Adams, S., and P. Burcher. 2014. In: *Feminist Phenomenology and Medicine*, edited by Kristin Zeiler and Lisa Käll, 69–80. Albany, NY: SUNY Press.

Leder, D. 1990. *The Absent Body.* Chicago, IL: University of Chicago Press.

Levinas, E. 1969. *Totality and Infinity: An Essay on Exteriority.* Translated by A. Lingis. Pennsylvania: Duquesne University Press.

LintottS., and M. Sander-Staudt, eds. 2012. *Philosophical Inquiries on Pregnancy, Childbirth and Mothering*. New York: Routledge.

Lundquist, C. 2008. "Being Torn: Toward a Phenomenology of Unwanted Pregnancy." *Hypatia* 23(3): 136–155.

Merleau-Ponty, M. 1962. *Phenomenology of Perception*. Translated by Colin Smith. London and New York: Routledge.

Michaels, M. 1996. "Other Mothers: Towards an Ethic of Postmaternal Practice." *Hypatia* 11(2): 49–70.

Mullin, A. 2005. *Reconceiving Pregnancy and Childcare: Ethics, Experience and Reproductive Labor*. New York: Cambridge University Press.

Narayan, U. 1995. "The 'Gift' of a Child: Commercial Surrogacy, Gift Surrogacy and Motherhood." In: *Expecting Trouble: Surrogacy, Fetal Abuse and New Reproductive Technologies*, edited by P. Boling, 177–202. Oxford: Westview Press.

Oliver, K. 2010. "Motherhood, Sexuality and Pregnant Embodiment: Twenty-Five Years of Gestation." *Hypatia* 25(4): 760–777.

Pande, A. 2009. "'It May Be Her Eggs But It's My Blood:' Surrogates and Everyday Forms of Kinship in India." *Qualitative Sociology* 32: 379–397.

Raymonds, J.G. 1993. *Women as Wombs: Reproductive Technologies and the Battle over Women's Freedom*. Melbourne, Australia: Spinifex Press.

Scarry, E. 1985. *The Body in Pain: The Making and Unmaking of the World*. New York: Oxford University Press.

Teman, E. 2009. "Embodying Surrogate Motherhood: Pregnancy as a Dyadic Body-project." *Body & Society* 15: 47–69.

Teman, E. 2010. *Birthing a Mother: The Surrogate Body and the Pregnant Self*. California: University California Press.

Toledano, S.J., and K. Zeiler. Forthcoming. "Hosting for the Others' Child? Relational Work and Embodied Responsibility in Altruistic Surrogate Motherhood." *Feminist Theory*.

Trobe, L. 2013. *A Womb with a View: America's Growing Public Interest in Pregnancy*. Santa Barbara, CA: Praeger.

Tyler, I. 2000. "Reframing Pregnant Embodiment." In: *Transformations: Thinking through Feminism*, edited by S. Ahmed, J. Kilby, C. Lury, M. McNeill and B. Skeggs. London: Routledge.

Van der Zalm, J. 2011. "Pregnancy." *Phenomenology Online: A Resource for Phenomenological Inquiry*. Available at: www.phenomenologyonline.com/sources/textorium/van-der-zalm-jeanne-pregnancy.

van Hooft, S. 2003. "Pain and Communication." *Medicine, Health Care and Philosophy* 6: 255–262.

Waldby, C. 2002. "Biomedicine, Tissue Transfer and Intercorporeality." *Feminist Theory* 3(3): 239–254.

Weiss, G. 1999. *Body Images: Embodiment as Intercorporeality*. New York: Routledge.

Welsh, T. 2008. "The Developing Body: A Reading of Merleau-Ponty's Conception of Women in the Sorbonne Lectures." In: *Intertwinings: Interdisciplinary Encounters with Merleau-Ponty*, edited by G. Weiss, 45–59. Albany, NY: SUNY Press.

Young, I.M. 1984. "Pregnant Embodiment: Subjectivity and Alienation." *Journal of Medicine and Philosophy* 9: 45–62.

Young, I.M. 2005. *On Female Body Experience: Throwing Like a Girl and Other Essays*. New York: Oxford University Press.

Zahavi, D. 2001. "Beyond Empathy: Phenomenological Approaches to Intersubjectivity." *Journal of Consciousness Studies* 8: 151–167.

Zahavi, D. 2011. "Intersubjectivity." In: *Routledge Companion to Phenomenology*, edited by S. Luft and O. Overgaard. London: Routledge. Available at: http://cfs.ku.dk/staff/zahavi-publications/Overgaard-Luft-Intersubjectivity-Routledge.pdf.

Zeiler, K. 2010. "A Phenomenological Analysis of Bodily Self-awareness in the Experience of Pain and Pleasure: On dys-appearance and eu-appearance." *Medicine, Healthcare and Philosophy* 13: 333–342.

Zeiler, K. 2014a. "Neither Property Right Nor Heroic Gift, Neither Sacrifice Nor Aporia: The Benefit of a Theoretical Lens of Sharing in Donation Ethics." *Medicine, Health Care and Philosophy* 17: 171–181.

Zeiler, K. 2014b. "A Philosophical Defense of the Idea that We Can Hold Each Other in Personhood: Intercorporeal Personhood in Dementia Care." *Medicine, Health Care and Philosophy* 17: 131–141.

8 Relational ontology and ethics in online organ solicitation

The problem of sharing one's body when being touched online

Kristin Zeiler

Introduction: Gail, Juan and Leigh Anne's story

"It's just amazing", reads the headline in *Chicago Sun Times* (Newbart 2007, 8). "In an extraordinary sacrifice, a man donates a kidney to a Northbrook woman, then his wife serves as a surrogate mother for her twins".

Gail Fink very much wanted to have a family. However, according to her doctors, her repeated IVF trials may have been what caused her kidney failure and she now needed a kidney transplant. Gail posted her story on MatchingDonors.com, a Massachusetts-based internet forum that links potential donors and recipients from all over the world. When Juan Uribe, a Hispanic Pentecostal minister in Texas, read Gail's post, his "heart went out to her", he told the newspaper and added that her "profile struck a chord with me" (ibid.). Juan donated one of his kidneys, and Gail recovered.

As a result, Gail could pursue her dream of starting a family. However, because of her medical condition, she had no viable eggs and undergoing a pregnancy would also be risky for her. After a friend volunteered to be an egg donor, Gail began her search for a surrogate mother. It was then that she turned to Leigh Anne, Juan's wife, and asked if Leigh Anne would consider serving as her surrogate mother, adding that she realized this might be asking too much. At first Leigh Anne responded that she did not think she could do it, but eventually she said yes.

As the newspaper recounts, Leigh Anne was formerly a linguist in the US army. When her Army unit was called up, she was spared a second tour in Iraq because Juan was recovering from a hernia at the site of the kidney transplant and could not take care of the couple's three children by himself. "A blessing", said Leigh Anne, explaining that she had prayed and reached the conclusion that "it seemed like I was supposed to do this" for Gail and her husband (ibid.). The second IVF attempt was successful and Leigh Anne carried two twin boys to term.

Gail, Juan and Leigh Anne's story can be read as going to the core of debates about gift-giving. One person presents a gift (in this case a kidney donation), a return gift is given (Leigh Anne remains in the USA, though one can discuss who gives this counter-gift), and as a result a new gift is given (the birth of twins for the intended parents). This chapter offers a different reading. Rather than being concerned with circles of gifts and counter-gifts, it explores how others' way of touching and affecting us can help shape our decisions, actions and existence, why the phenomenon of touching and being touched needs to be acknowledged in ethics and why it evokes fundamental concerns in online organ solicitation.

The chapter turns to phenomenological philosophy and to the phenomenological notion of giving-through-sharing that has been used in order to explore whether and how the donation of an organ (the giving) can be understood as an expression of the connectedness and continuity between the self and the other (the sharing), which is the very precondition of the self as embodied and situated in a world and in relation to others in phenomenological reasoning (Zeiler 2014b). As described by Fredrik Svenaeus in this volume, phenomenological philosophy studies philosophical questions by proceeding from an analysis of lived experience. When exploring and seeking to understand ontological issues, the focus is on the meaning structures of the everyday world, on that which is often referred to as our being-in-the-world. This is also my starting point. However, my present interest is in what can be labelled as relational ontology, i.e. how that which is, is relationally formed, and how some such formations are ethically more problematic than others. In this way, I want to offer a phenomenological approach to the ethics of online organ solicitation. While the chapter starts from an understanding of giving-through-sharing as a condition for human existence and co-existence, the focus is on the affective, formative and potentially also ethically problematic dimensions of this sharing.

The chapter draws upon Maurice Merleau-Ponty's (2006) phenomenological work when addressing the issue of being touched online, and seeks to "think with touch" (Puig de la Bellacasa 2009) in order understand vision that touches and moves us in the case of online organ solicitation. It engages with the ancient myth of Psyche and Cupid, and with the work of Rosalyn Diprose (2006) in order to discuss how the social expression and sharing of meaning through processes of touching and being touched can co-constitute us as human beings, why being able to be touched by the other is ethically positive and yet a reason for concern in relation to online organ solicitation. First, however, the chapter contrasts ethical concerns over online organ solicitation and donation with established ethical rationales for post-mortem and live donations to unknown second parties on the one hand and live donations to family-members and friends on the other. It examines how online organ solicitation and directed donation falls between common ways of thinking about donation ethics, and why online organ solicitation and the subsequent donation should evoke more concerns than those about how donation queues may be side-stepped.

Online organ solicitation

MatchingDonors.com is one of the largest online organ solicitation sites worldwide, although others also exist, such as FloodSisters.org. These websites have been launched from different states of the USA, which evokes questions as to the cultural context and legal jurisdiction in which launching an online organ solicitation site may be perceived as a possibility. Although prospective donors from all over the world are welcome to log in, recipients at MatchingDonors.com must be residents of the USA or the UK. Thus, the donations are not for the benefit of everyone. A study has also shown that a higher proportion of those soliciting kidneys online in the USA were employed or white than the proportion on the general waiting list (Rodrigue *et al.* 2008).

Few studies have investigated why people seeking organ transplantation go online. In one such case, respondents explained that they had not been able to find a match through their "face-to-face networks" (Costello and Murillo 2014). Turning to the internet was described as a way to widen that network, and as less difficult emotionally than asking others to consider donating face-to-face. Marketing oneself was also described as part of the process, as was expressing oneself in positive terms (ibid.). Another study showed that individuals who provided personal information such as a photograph, place of residence, age, blood type and history of dialysis had a higher success rate in terms of attracting potential donors for compatibility testing after online solicitation on Facebook (Chang *et al.* 2013).

The phenomenon of online organ solicitation can be compared to other online activities, such as mail-order brides or fundraising for communities struck by natural disasters or war. By contrast, however, online organ solicitation does not seek financial aid for anyone and the benefactor is a specific individual, not a group or a community. The idea seems not to be to get to know and become emotionally close to one other person (as in the case of the mail-order bride) but to ask for help from anyone.

Finally, online solicitation is only possible because ours is a time when some people can connect across space and time via the internet. On the one hand, virtual communities may be seen as open and fluid, and online solicitation via Facebook, chat rooms and websites can allow for patient agency in new ways. On the other hand, such agency is unequally distributed. By posting her or his story, any individual may elicit responses from any other, and there is no formal hierarchy in how this is done (at least not on Facebook). Nevertheless, the online forum's non-hierarchy is a chimera. Individuals capable of writing and posting a telling and appealing story, and having the appropriate skill and access to the internet, will have an advantage over others.

Why online organ solicitation doesn't correspond to established donation ethics

Online organ solicitation and the subsequent donation is directed towards a specific other of the donor's own choosing, which makes it similar to live donation to known others; yet the receiver has no prior relation to the donor, as in the case of post-mortem organ donation and live organ donation to unknown others.

The specificity of this donation can be brought out by way of contrast, first with organ donation to unknown others. Live bodily donation to unknown others differs in many ways from the post-mortem case, but both donations take place between individuals who do *not* know each other and without the donor having decision-making authority as regards who the recipient(s) shall be. Donors can therefore qualify as impartial agents (having no prior relation to the recipient) and recipients can be said to have fair access to donated material according to their place on the local hospital's donor list (even though one may discuss the criteria for being put high on this list). The ethical rationale of post-mortem and live donation to unknown others can qualify as one of "impartial altruism", where people act for the benefit of another irrespective of previous knowledge of the identity of that person (McGee 2005).

The case of live donation to family-members or friends is different. Whether this donation is motivated out of love, obligation, or for other reasons, the rationale for it rests with a pre-existing relationship. Donors and recipients share a history that can inform the wish to donate. In fact, living donation has been described as "partial" and "'unfortunate' in that it favors some people over others" (Hilhurst *et al.* 2005, 1473). However, while this partial donation jeopardizes justice-as-fair-access based on one's place on a donor list, it is often understood as ethically acceptable if donors have been adequately informed about alternatives, have thought through the decision to donate and are not socially pressured into donating. Responding to the needs of family-members and friends has been seen as partial as well as ethically valuable: as family-members or friends, donors may have felt emotional or moral commitments to the recipients that made them want to act in this way (Crouch and Elliot 1999).

The two different ethical rationales include two distinct ways of thinking about the relation between self and other. The first ethical rationale of donation to unknown others, that of impartial altruism, is compatible with the idea that impartial giving has genuine moral worth because it does not bestow special weight on one's own interests, preferences or desires any more than on someone else's, i.e. one should not treat family-members or friends any differently than others. Against this impartiality position, it has been held that a world in which we accord everyone the same consideration would not result in a "big happy family" but would leave us devoid of the affection of our children, partners or friends because they would cease being special to us (Cottingham 1983, 90). The second ethical rationale of donation to family-members and friends, that of allowing donations to specific others, hence, partiality, belongs to ethical approaches that focus on emotional and moral commitments to others with whom we share our lives.

However, scholars who argue for the importance of acknowledging the special bond between family-members and friends and the particular form of self-referential altruism that may accompany it (I donate to my family-members or friends because of our connection over time), can still hold that *others* to whom we have no such special relation fall outside the scope of this kind of altruism. To donate to someone whose story resonates with us is not to donate impartially, nor is it to follow the self-referential altruism that builds on a pre-existing relation.

Online organ solicitation and directed donation have been criticized for being susceptible to beauty-, social-capital-, or financial-capital-related inequalities. Scholars have pointed to the risk of a "beauty contest" in which the individual with the most appealing story or the most photogenic face will attract donors at the expense of others (Steinbrook 2005; Truog 2005). Similarly, online donation has been faulted for allowing the flourishing of group bias where donors may donate in particular ways based on racial or ideological preferences (Neidich *et al.* 2012). Furthermore, concerns have been raised that transnational bodily exchanges of this kind may be easier for those with greater or the right linguistic competence and the experience of going abroad, and can involve costs (even if it does not imply an illicit financial reward for donors) that only some will be able to afford.

At the heart of these criticisms is a concern for fairness, which proponents of the online organ solicitation seek to rebut. They argue that recipients on waiting lists are not negatively affected by having to wait longer because of the introduction of online solicitation (the assumption being that donors who volunteer via websites would not have donated to unknown others in other ways, see Truog 2005), and that living donations to known others such as family-members or friends are already based on a form of unfairness "resulting from chance" (since not everyone has family-members or friends who can and are willing to donate). It has been claimed that online solicitation helps "to offset inequity introduced by chance" (Wright and Campbell 2006, 5).

Since these donations are unusual (100 donations were arranged via MatchingDonors.com in the US during a seven-year period according to the website's newsletter in 2011, see Neidich *et al.* 2012), the consequences for the waiting list may not be great, even if these donors might have considered donating to unknown others on a donation list instead, and although the consequences for each individual who does not receive a kidney quickly or at all can still be very serious. Still, for those with a less consequentialist leaning, the issue is whether organ solicitation can be ethically justified as a means of increasing organ donation regardless of how common it is.

Online organ solicitation and directed donation can be viewed as problematic when allowing individuals to side-step donation queues (an issue of justice) without having "the right kind" of partiality (such as family or friendship relations over time). Yet something more is going on. In commenting on the phenomenon of online organ solicitation, Ellen McGee (2005) suggests that one alternative may be to allow for stories that motivate donation, but not for potential donors to decide to whom to donate. Pictures and stories seem to have a motivating function, and empathic responses that they elicit can be directed into the established organ donation system rather than being banned.

This, however, would break the link between recipients and donors on which online organ solicitation seems to depend; the potential donors would no longer be responding and donating to a specific visual–textual other of their own choosing.

McGee sees this link as ethically troublesome. While we may agree, it is not only because of justice concerns but for other fundamental reasons that can best be spelled out by exploring the phenomenon of being touched by another. A reading of the ancient myth of Psyche and Cupid can illustrate the issue (Apuleius 1989).

Psyche's dilemma

In the myth, Psyche is a princess who draws upon herself the wrath of Aphrodite, the goddess of love and beauty, by unintentionally being compared to her. Aphrodite sends her son Cupid to revenge herself, but as the story unfolds, Cupid and Psyche become lovers. However, while Psyche spends her days in a beautiful castle, with invisible servants and all the luxuries she could ever want, and her nights with Cupid, he never tells her who he is but rather explains that she must never see him in the light. Each morning before daybreak, Cupid leaves Psyche and does not return until night. And as time goes on, Psyche starts to desire to see him. This yearning is also driven by her sisters' suspicious questioning. Who is this being with whom Psyche lives? Torn between her wish to heed Cupid's warning and her desire to see him, Psyche decides to steal a glimpse of her loved one, and so, one night, she lights a candle, rendering him visible.

In a common reading, the myth underlines the link between visibility and belief, where seeing is believing and vision implies revelation. If Psyche faces a dilemma, it is a dilemma that brings to light the uncertainty over what role to attribute to sight and visibility in meaning-making and for action. In online solicitation, this uncertainty can be articulated when individuals see the visual–textual other presented before them as they consider donation, because they have been touched by the photo and the story, while at the same time being concerned that there are issues with this donation – issues that have to do with the role of visibility for how we act towards others.

However, the myth also allows for another reading, which I see as more productive for my current concern. Thinking back to the myth, Psyche has already been touched by Cupid before seeing him, and this may well have contributed to her actions. While this is typically not the case for organ donors and solicitors online, this *being touched beforehand* still offers a key to the analysis of the ethical problematic of online solicitation.

The word touch has ambiguous meanings and two partially overlapping understandings can be distinguished: the sense of touch and being touched emotionally (as in touch that affects us). However, while much can be said about the interrelation between these two (being touched emotionally can take place with or without physical touch, and being touched emotionally can also have corporeal, physical effects: my heart beats faster and my attention becomes focused on – or I turn away from – that which touches me emotionally), my present focus is on how we have, all of us, been touched by others, just as Psyche was touched and affected by Cupid and by others such as her sisters before she lit the candle.

How we have been touched by others can orient us in space and make us disposed to act in particular ways. A phenomenological explication of this latter phenomenon, combined with María Puig de la Bellacasa's (2009, 298) call to "think with touch" will illuminate the ethical problematic of online organ solicitation and directed donation.

A phenomenology of giving-through-sharing

In *Phenomenology of Perception*, Maurice Merleau-Ponty (2006) argues that it is because we inhabit bodies that pre-reflectively open up a world of meaning to us that we can approach things and people through perception, action and language. The body, according to this reasoning, is my lived relation to a world immersed in meaning, which is opened up to me through my bodily senses and made meaningful to me in interactions with others. This is a shared world, steeped in cultural significance, and shaped, made meaningful and rendered familiar to me by others. In this sense, I am given the world, and myself, in relations with others.

Consider how Merleau-Ponty (2006, 419) uses the notion of being given, when he writes that the

> central phenomenon, at the root of both my subjectivity and my transcendence towards others, consists in my being given to myself. *I am given*, that is, I find myself already situated and involved in a physical and social world – *I am given to myself*, which means that this situation is never hidden from me, it is never round about me as an alien necessity, and I am never in effect enclosed in it like an object in a box.

To be given to oneself is a description of the human life condition. I am not separated from others and the world. However, if I am given the world and myself in relations with others, then this takes place through a basic and dynamic sharing of our being-in-the-world. In other words, the giving at stake is primarily not that in which I give *away* something to others for their keeping, but a *giving-through-sharing* that brings out the basic connectedness between self and other (Zeiler 2014a, 2014b).

The phenomenon of giving-through-sharing can be exemplified in cases where we have thought through how to "give" the world to others as intelligible, as when seeking to make someone comfortable in a new situation by showing her or him how to act after having reflected upon how best to do so. More commonly, we may give by sharing our mode of being-in-the-world without thinking about how we do so, or that we are doing it. Such pre-reflective giving-through-sharing takes place when we "just" act in a particular way and when someone else starts to act the same way by mimicking our behaviour, or our ways of acting or interacting. In this way, we may "give" a certain way of being-in-the-world to our children – by sharing our own being-in-the-world with them. As another example, Gail Weiss (1999, 2) discusses how body images are "construed through a series of corporeal exchanges that take place both within and outside of specific bodies" in engagement with others. While my body image may be seen as personal, it is continuously formed in interactions with others, hence it is never only personal. By sharing – and not always intentionally so – our patterns of behaviour or ways of understanding or feeling for something, our being-in-the-world can shape the being-in-the-world of others. We "give" the world as meaningful to others by "sharing" it. We give-through-sharing.

Sharing meaning together with others can give rise to a familiarity that can be understood in terms of a sense of belonging where I "feel at home" in the world and which typically is not the result of a conscious decision. Instead, as put by Rosalyn Diprose (2006, 382–383), "meaning comes to me through habituated dwelling with other bodies and this incarnation, sharing, and expression of meaning is affective, ambiguous and transformative". The social expression of meaning in interactions with others can inform our bodily way of being, even when we do not think about it, and this sharing can result in a sense of affinity with some people more than others.

At stake is a philosophical perspective that brings to light how bodily subjects are constantly formed in relation to each other, whether we like it or not, how the self is not isolated from others.[1] Emphasis is put on embodied interaction and connectedness between subject and object, and this becomes particularly clear in Merleau-Ponty's analysis of the senses of touch and vision.

To think with touch

It has been suggested that to "think with touch has a potential to inspire a sense of connectedness that can problematize abstractions and … disengaged distances" between subjects and objects (Puig de la Bellacasa 2009, 298, 299). For Merleau-Ponty, to think with touch in relation to vision affirms the embodied and situated character of both of these senses. On the one hand, he insists that it is misleading to consider the senses as sharply separated from each other. They are all interconnected in my body; each sense involves a complex of sensations, and together they constitute perception. On the other hand, he holds that the sense of touch offers less of an illusion of non-situatedness than vision and makes clear how the body opens up the world to us.

The latter makes it helpful to think with touch in order to think the connectedness between subject and object. Referring to the experience of one's right hand touching the left, or the handshake, Merleau-Ponty observes that to be touching is also to be touched, although these two aspects never fully coincide. For him, this shows how the body mediates the relation between subject and object, being both subject and object, sentient and sensed. The connectedness between subject and object in the case of touching hands reminds us of how our experience of our own bodies is formed in relation to others and to the world as co-constitution, that is, we may touch others and objects in the world and they may touch us in ways that form our own very mode of touching (compare Käll 2009). As an example, I may experience the other's hand that squeezes mine in a handshake as firm or painful, and how I experience this can form my way of seeking to squeeze back or withdraw in pain. How the other touches me can form my mode of touching, how specific others have shaken our hands in the past may well inform how we greet them in the present.

The case of touch, being touched and touching, opens up for analysis how bodily subjects form each other in relations and within specific historical and social fields, and how the phenomenon of being touched in the past can feed into the present. However, while Merleau-Ponty focuses on the sense of touch, the points I want to make rest with the ambiguous meanings of touch (as in the interplay between the sense of touch and being touched emotionally), with how being touched can affect and form us and with the phenomenon of touching vision.

Two points can be made based on this reasoning. First, if vision is understood according to the model of touch, as suggested by Merleau-Ponty, the connectedness between the self that sees, others and the world that are seen, and others who see me becomes clearer. My image of myself is formed by others' communicated perceptions of me which in turn can inform how I see myself and them. I am not separated from others and the world, but connected with them. And it is not only my body image that is formed in corporeal exchanges, but habituated dwelling with some specific others can give rise to a familiarity where I may feel more at home with some people than others. I may experience a sense of affinity with some people more than others because of a basic sharing of meaning, because of how I have been seen by, touched by and familiarized with them, and this is not optional but a condition of existence. Second, touch, here, need not be limited to physical touch as in the handshake. The idea is rather that to think with touch helps us bring to light the formative, affective and pre-reflective aspects of human co-existence including how the social expression and sharing of meaning through processes of touching and being touched, physically or emotionally, can co-constitute us as human beings. How we have been touched beforehand can help form our pre-reflective ways of being-in-the-world, to put it in phenomenological terms. In this way, to think with touch can help bring to light the formative dimension of the phenomenon of giving-through-sharing as a human life condition, and this matters for the discussion of relational ontology and ethics in the online organ solicitation case.

Being touched online

To be touched by another individual, physically as well as online, implies exposure. While we do not experience the other's eyes meeting ours via websites and online networks as when eyes meet or we touch in everyday encounters, the visual–textual exposition of the other on the screen does render her or him visible in this medium. And that result may affect us. At the same time, of course, and in contrast to physical hand-to-hand touching, there is no immediate reversibility between touching and being touched in the case of being touched online. If the individual in need of an organ donation is being touched by our response when touching us, then this reversibility is unsure, perhaps delayed in time and can involve a frustrating wait. While connection online can allow for the experience of presence or co-presence online, it can also lead to an experience of absence when others do not respond to our online feeds.

We may also be more anonymous online. While we may be touched by the visual–textual other, the online forum offers a distance to the organ solicitor that doesn't exist if a person with kidney failure asks us to donate in a face-to-face encounter. In the former case, we may simply turn off the computer. Despite this, part of the allure of what may be called "touching vision online" may reside in how those who are geographically distant others may come to be experienced as present. In contrast to the spatio-temporal constriction that phenomenologists have explored in relation to pain, where I cannot but attend to my bodily discomfort, here and now (Leder 1990), the online experience can be characterized by both a spatio-temporal constriction in the sense that I experience the geographically distant other as present, in real time, *and* an expansion of my here-and-now by making it present online for those who can connect through this medium. It has also been suggested that touching images can push the viewer close to that which or who we see in a way that makes the viewer relinquish "her own sense of separateness from the image", as when being immersed in a film (Marks 2000, 124). While there may be variations in how different media do this and a variation in terms of how likely we are to be pushed in this way, some images and texts seem capable of moving some of us considerably.[2]

Now, the giving-through-sharing of social meaning explained how we may – through words and deeds – contribute to others' sense of familiarity and belonging to a particular social world by how we share our mode of being. Diprose put this well when explaining that this

> sense of belonging is not located in a table of shared values and social meanings that I *reflect* upon or that I use to identify with and recognize in others; rather this familiarity is located in my body as an atmosphere that informs how I perceive the world as I live through it.
>
> (Diprose 2006, 382)

My unique bodily existence is informed by for example others' understandings of bodies and of how to interact with specific bodily others and the world. Others way of giving me the world by sharing it makes it familiar to me, and through mimicking others' ways of acting, interacting, thinking and feeling I can come to incorporate parts of their modes of being-in-the-world. Furthermore, if some such ways of acting, interacting, thinking or feeling are repeated over time, they can become part of my habitual style of being and be what I "just" do, or how I "just" react to certain situations, without thinking about this.

This is not to say that we simply adjust to the way of being of others. The sharing of meaning is dynamic and potentially transformative, and may lead us to act contrary to our habitual style of being. However, depending on how others have co-shaped our world, perceptions of others as individuals whom we can relate to and respond to can be formed by habituated ways of engaging with others. Whether responding to the other's calls for help online by volunteering as a donor stands forth *as for me* may depend on my particular bodily style of being, my habituated way of engaging with others, my body's capacities and the collective familiar modes of responding to others' calls that may have become part of my pattern of acting and interacting.

This is also what I want to spell out with the language of touch and the idea of touching vision: there is a connectedness between self and other, where self and other form one another. The way others touch me can form my way of touching them and others, and we may be more likely to be touched and affected by others that we experience as familiar or that "resonate" with us as Juan put it when describing why he donated to Gail. Who we may be likely to resonate with can be informed by the phenomenon of being touched beforehand and in this sense, social life has its ethically problematic aspects. How we "just" respond to others may depend upon the social meanings attributed to specific bodily others, without us even being reflectively aware of it, and of how others' ways of touching us may have oriented us in space so that in the future we are more likely to be touched by some individuals than others. The social meanings that inform our sense of belonging may make us more likely to be touched by individuals with whom we pre-reflectively feel at home. This "pre-reflective sense of belonging" can contribute to or even prolong discrimination (Diprose 2006, 383) making it an ethical concern, and this is the reason why the problem with online corporeal donation goes deeper than how donations may contribute to inequalities with regard to waiting lists. It concerns the conditions for being touched by the needs of others and being moved to take action. This is an ethical issue, and it underscores that ethics can preferably be understood to include "the problem of what constitutes one's habitat, the problematic of corporeal self-formation in relation to other social beings and within the laws and discourses that regulate those relations" (Diprose 2005, 239).

To think with touch in this way makes clear the need for a continuous critical examination of how we come to perceive each other, how we may be touched by one another and how we may be less inclined to be touched by certain others. And to return to the case of Psyche, she has touched and been touched by Cupid before seeing him, but her existence is not only shared with him but also with her sisters. Whether lighting the candle stands forth as a viable possibility for her may be informed by her relation to them – and how they and their questioning affect her. This is not to say that she is not responsible for her action, but rather to emphasize the sociality of what we may come to perceive as possible routes of action. In a related way, even if potential organ donors and prospective recipients do not know each other beforehand, whether donors become touched online can hinge on how they have already been touched by others and how they remain open to being altered by others.

An ethics of touch

Merleau-Ponty emphasizes that my bodily existence is open to others who are different from me, and that this makes the expression of social meaning dynamic and subject to change. While he did not elaborate an ethics based on his reasoning (although he suggested that this could be done), it could be claimed that if there is an ethical challenge in Merleau-Ponty's work, it is to remain open to being affected and transformed in encounters with others. In this way, whether or not I become touched by others may be restricted by how I have already been touched by others in the past, by the sedimentation of shared meanings that inform my bodily way of being-in-the-world, but "it would be unethical if I shut out the unfamiliar through vilification or violence as a matter of personal or political policy" (Diprose 2006, 386).

What makes online solicitation and directed donation potentially troubling is that being touched online typically is a pre-reflective phenomenon even though we may try to rationalize it at a later stage. We "just" become touched by some people more than others, and those we are touched by may be the ones we feel "at home" with, who resemble us or those who we care for and love in ways that, from another perspective, cannot qualify as fair. However, while online solicitation and directed donation appear dependent on the phenomenon of being touched beforehand, it would be misleading to label this an ethical problem.

What may be called an ethics of touch presupposes the ability to be touched by others.[3] Such an ethics would affirm the connectedness between self and other as a condition for being touched at all, and would require a critical analysis of whether, in which way, and by whom we may be touched online and an acknowledgement that one should strive to remain open and "touchable" also by those we may at first perceive as strangers. As a basis for ethics, the ability to be touched, at all, is crucial – even if this is not to say that touch as such is ethical (and there may indeed be various forms of touch, from the caress to the blow).

On the one hand, we can be touched by others because of the basic openness and connectedness between self and other, and when seeing the other in pain, when listening to another's story, we may be touched and feel called upon to respond to this individual because of how we *have already been touched by others.* We already take part in a shared meaning-making, and this also allows short and fragmentary stories of living with pain to say something to us. Regardless of why potential donors go online, they can be touched there because they have already been gripped by shared human existence and common suffering.

This can be further explained via Jean-Luc Nancy's (2012) discussion of touch and community, where he holds that community is commonly thought of in terms of coalescence around a fixed identity or essence, as common-being in terms of a presumed unity. Nancy considers these nostalgic illusions that downplay the singularity, ineradicable otherness and finitude of each of us when we turn towards others for support, help or confirmation. For him, this conception of community is problematic and underlies present-day conflicts where individuals identify with a community based on ideas of unity and stand in opposition to other communities. The same notion could also drive group-based preferences regarding organ donation.

Nancy's alternative is to understand community as something that exists through engagement of singular beings exposed to each other. As singular beings, he holds, we share finitude, the condition of being-with-others, and being born into a world that others make meaningful for us. For this reason, in Nancy's vocabulary, singular beings are always plural, and community is where singular plural beings are exposed to each other and engage in ever-incomplete sharing of meaning – incomplete in the sense that it is on-going and never fully within someone's "control". Nancy is concerned with the circulation of meaning or signification, how meaning is created, shared out and divided between different singular beings, and his conception of community seeks to emphasize the ontological necessity of the relational. What we share is not a presumed unity or property but the conditions that allow sharing: exposure to each other by virtue of our bodies that allow us to come into contact and touch each other.

This alternative understanding of community in which individuals are understood as engaged in an incomplete sharing of meaning, allows for a shift in focus from groups of different kinds to encounters between singular beings. Such encounters, according to Nancy, imply exposure. We can be affected by each other without being able to fully know each other's suffering. We may not have so much in common, but *we are* in common, exposed to each other. We are continuously touched by each other, and this forms singular plural existence, and points to the depth of our engagement with each other whether we like it or not.

On the other hand, we may not be touched by all others in the same way. This brings us back to the argument within this chapter. We are always-already touched by others and in this sense we are continuously, dynamically and relationally formed. We form each other by touching each other and sharing our being-in-the-world, *and* this enables some of us to be touched online, by some and not others.

When Leigh Anne goes online, she exposes herself to others. She renders herself visible and calls for help. Juan sees her advertisement online, is touched and ultimately responds by donating.[4] While the ability to be touched by the other should be seen as a condition for ethics and something to be striven for, how we are touched by others, who touches us and who doesn't should also be crucial concerns. Ethically speaking, online organ solicitation evokes not only concerns about side-stepping donation queues, but also basic concerns about the problematic of asymmetrically shared, pre-reflective, and affective meaning-making in social life, and potential implications of this for the practice of online organ solicitation and subsequent directed donation. It evokes concerns about the ethically problematic sides of the basic openness between self and other that makes possible this shared, pre-reflective, affective and asymmetrical meaning-making. And rather than being put aside as pre-ethical, that is, as not ethical but motivating the emergence of ethical reflection, such meaning-making needs to be part of the ethical examination. In this way, the phenomenon of online organ solicitation should concern us – beyond the issue of donation queues being side-stepped.

Acknowledgements

I wish to thank the participants at the symposium *Sharing Bodies within and across Borders*, and Fredrik Svenaeus in particular, for comments on an earlier version of this text. This research is part of my work as *Pro Futura Scientia* Fellow at the Swedish Collegium for Advanced Study (SCAS), Uppsala University, financially supported by SCAS and *Riksbankens Jubileumsfond*.

Notes

1 Similarities and differences involved in the sharing of embodied meaning patterns that are found in many everyday encounters and in the sharing of organs have been explored elsewhere (see Zeiler 2014b). The present discussion restricts itself to phenomenological thinking on touch, vision and embodied interaction, and I will therefore not enter the discussion about such similarities and differences.

2 It may seem odd to turn to an account of embodiment such as Merleau-Ponty's, and to his discussion of the sense of touch, in order to explore what may be perceived as a rather disembodied case of being touched online, but an analysis of the online phenomenon benefits from thinking through embodiment. The physical and emotional dimensions of touch can intermingle in both physical and online cases of being touched by the other, but for my present reasoning, the point of thinking with touch is to explore the formative dimension of our being-in-the-world with others.

3 What is here referred to as an ethics of touch overlaps with what might be called an ethics of empathy (in the sense of feeling with others). In both cases, the question of how we may do good towards others is considered by stressing emotions that can tie us together. The term an ethics of touch, however, by way of association, can help us think through the corporeal dimension of how we may be touched by, and feel-with, another. Rather than seeing this as a problem when examining the phenomenon of being touched online, one should recall that human existence is always embodied, and that our concrete embodiment can shape those we can be emotionally touched by – even online.

4 In addition to the ethical issues raised by this form of donation, one might ask if there is not something ethically disturbing when or if a health care system is dependent on people begging for organ donation in front of strangers, in the form of online organ solicitation. Furthermore, touching vision could lead to self-sacrificing acts that need to be examined.

References

Apuleius. 1989. *Metamorphoses (The Golden Ass), volume II.* Translated by J.A. Hanson. Cambridge, MA, and London: Harvard University Press.

Chang, A., AndersonE.E., Turner, H.T., Shoham, D., Hou, S.H., and M. Grams. 2013. "Identifying Potential Kidney Donors Using Social Networking Websites." *Clinical Transplantation* 27: E320–E326.

Costello, K.L. and A.P. Murillo. 2014. "'I Want Your Kidney!' Information Seeking, Sharing, and Disclosure when Soliciting a Kidney Donor Online." *Patient Education and Counseling* 94: 423–426.

Cottingham, J. 1983. "Ethics and Impartiality." *Philosophical Studies* 43: 83–99.

Crouch, R.A. and C. Elliot. 1999. "Moral Agency and the Family: The Case of Living Related Organ Transplantation." *Cambridge Quarterly of Healthcare Ethics* 8(3): 275–287.

Diprose, R. 2005. "A 'Genethics' that Makes Sense: Take Two." In*: Ethics of the Body: Postconventional Challenges*, edited by M. Shildrick and R. Mykitiuk, 237–258. Cambridge, MA: The MIT Press.

Diprose, R. 2006. "Community of Bodies: From Modification to Violence." *Continuum: Journal of Media & Cultural Studies* 19(3): 381–392.

Hilhurst, M.T., Kranenburg, L.W., Zuidema, W., Weimar, W., Ijzermans, J.N.M., Passchier, J. and J.J.V. Busschbach. 2005. "Altruistic Living Kidney Donation Challenges Psychosocial Research and Policy: A Response to Previous Articles." *Transplantation* 79(11): 1470–1474.

Käll, L.F. 2009. "A Being of Two Leaves – On the Founding Significance of the Lived Body." In: *Body Claims*, edited by J. Bromseth, L.F. Käll and K. Mattson, 110–133. Uppsala: Uppsala Universitet.

Leder, D. 1990. *The Absent Body.* Chicago and London: The University of Chicago Press.

Marks, L.U. 2000. *The Skin of the Film: Intercultural Cinema, Embodiment and the Senses.* Durham, NC and London: Duke University Press.

McGee, E. 2005. "Using Personal Narratives to Encourage Organ Donation." *American Journal of Bioethics* 5(4): 19–20.

Merleau-Ponty, M. 2006. *Phenomenology of Perception*. London: Routledge.

Nancy, J.-L. 2012. *The Inoperative Community*, edited by P. Connor. Mineapolis: University of Minnesota Press.

Neidich, E.M., Neidich, A.B., Cooper, J.T., and K.A. Bramstedt. 2012. "The Ethical Complexities of Online Organ Solicitation via Donor–Patient Websites: Avoiding the 'Beauty Contest'." *American Journal of Transplantation* 12: 43–47.

Newbart, D. 2007. "The Greatest Gift." *Chicago Sun Times*, December 25.

Puig de la Bellacasa, M. 2009. "Touching Technologies, Touching Vision. The Reclaiming of Sensorial Experience and the Politics of Speculative Thinking." *Subjectivity* 28: 297–315.

Rodrigue J.R., Antonellis, T., Mandelbrot, D.A., and D.W. Hanto. 2008. "Web-based Requests for Living Organ Donors: Who Are the Solicitors?" *Clinical Transplantation* 22: 749–753.

Steinbrook, R. 2005. "Public Solicitation of Organ Donors." *New England Journal of Medicine* 353(3): 441–444.

Truog, R.D. 2005. "The Ethics of Organ Donation by Living Donors." *New England Journal of Medicine* 353(3): 444–446.

Weiss, G. 1999. *Body Images: Embodiment as Intercorporeality.* New York: Routledge.

Wright, L. and M. Campbell. 2006. "Soliciting Kidneys on Web Sites: Is It Fair?" *Seminars in Dialysis* 19(1): 5–7.

Zeiler, K. 2014a. "Neither Property Right nor Heroic Gift, neither Sacrifice nor Aporia: the Benefit of the Theoretical Lens of Sharing in Donation Ethics." *Medicine, Health Care and Philosophy* 17(2): 171–181.

Zeiler, K. 2014b. "A Phenomenological Approach to the Ethics of Transplantation Medicine: Sociality and Sharing when Living-with and Dying-with Others." *Theoretical Medicine and Bioethics* 35: 369–388.

9 The transplant imaginary and its postcolonial hauntings

Donna McCormack

Transplant imaginaries, or haunting histories

> It is a case of haunting, a story about what happens when we admit the ghost – that special instance of the merging of the visible and the invisible, the dead and the living, the past and the present – into the making of worldly relations and into the making of our accounts of the world. It is a case of the difference it makes to start with the marginal, with what we normally exclude or banish, or, more commonly, with what we never even notice.
>
> (Gordon 2008, 24–25)

> I accepted the kidney. Or is it maybe the kidney that ended up integrating me into it and digesting, filtering, and pissing out all my tormented feelings? Without rejecting the organ, without failure. A mutual assimilation and truce … But this tolerance couldn't keep me from thinking that with this organ, surgery had implanted in me two seeds of strangeness, of difference: the other sex and another "race."
>
> (Mokeddem 1998, 21)

Transplant imaginaries evoke the often unspeakable histories that haunt organ transplantation. As Avery Gordon intimates, such hauntings open up the possibility of getting close to the silenced or unspoken experiences that blur the distinctions between one's own body and that of an other, "the dead and the living, the past and the present". In his philosophical reflections on his own experience of a heart transplant, Jean-Luc Nancy describes how his failing heart was the site and source of intrusion: "My heart became my stranger: strange precisely because it was inside. The strangeness could only come from outside because it surged up first on the inside" (Nancy 2008, 163–164). The imminent failure of *his* heart called for its extrusion as it no longer maintained the self and was thus potentially deadly to the self. Intrusion of a sense of otherness comes not from the outside – as is commonly figured in relation to medical interventions and, of course, migration across borders. Rather his *own* heart came to feel – as in came to be experienced as – other, strange and dangerous. Survival was only possible through the introduction to the self of this supposedly alien object: a heart that *belonged* to an other. An other's heart that was strange to the self was thus willingly taken into his body and yet still lived as an intrusion, as a crossing of the hitherto immutable border between self and other. Nancy's sense of self and of relationality with this other is simultaneously intimate and strange. He is of the other without being other, and still his self, and yet an altered post-transplant self. The other is integral to and constitutive of a sense of (a post-transplant) self, yet absent and ever elusive. Here, the other is a haunting presence, simultaneously dead and alive, of the self and the other, and proximal and distant.

For Nancy, transplantation evokes concerns regarding ethical responsibility and relationality through difference. I want to expand on Nancy's reference to racialized, sexed and national difference by examining Malika Mokeddem's formulation of organ transplantation as implanting in the recipient "seeds of strangeness, of difference".[1] In so doing, I suggest that what it means to move organs from one body to another is intimately tied to anxieties concerning migrations across not only bodily boundaries but also national borders. It is the suturing of transplantation to anxieties around otherness and difference that I am concerned with in this article. More specifically, I am interested in how narratives of organ transplantation evoke broader socio-political and ethical concerns around encounters between self and other. Particularly, how they engage the contemporary issue of migration, raising questions about how bodily differences are produced as hierarchical. I explore organ transplantation and its associated socio-political problematics to examine how both national narratives and transplant teams demand a normative structure of time and selfhood. Indeed, I argue that transplantation and migration disrupt linear temporalities and the dominant notion of selfhood as an individual and disembodied state. Haunted by histories that the post-independent nation tries to silence and by the presence of an organ that is a reminder of the absence of the donor, national narratives and organ recipients coincide to convey a disruption, a "seething presence" (Gordon 2008, 8), that will not allow the self or the nation to continue on as if the past could be forgotten. Indeed, I address what it means to remember that which is absent, and analyse how a haunting absence – what Mokeddem (1998, 65) calls a "presence–absence" – is a form of remembering anonymous, silenced and unspoken histories.[2] In other words, I argue that in a shared cultural imaginary, organ donation is a nexus for the problematics of embodied difference across national and individual boundaries and a haunting absence reminding us of what we do not want to, refuse to or cannot remember.

The focus of this chapter is what could be described as a transplant imaginary. To a certain extent such a concept is inseparable from a broader scientific or biotechnological imaginary. Anneke Smelik (2010, 10) describes how the scientific imaginary raises "critical and ethical issues about contemporary science", specifically concerning "new technologies in science" (ibid., 10–11). Jackie Stacey argues in *The Cinematic Life of the Gene* that "the genetic imaginary constitutes a set of very tangible anxieties surrounding the reconfiguration of the human body" (Stacey 2010, 8). She adds that this genetic landscape could be described as "the mise-en-scène of these anxieties, a fantasy landscape inhabited by artificial bodies that disturb the conventional teleologies of gender, reproduction, racialization and heterosexual kinship" (ibid.). I also follow on from Lisa Cartwright's *Screening the Body* where she examines how fictional texts are "a part of the social apparatus through which Western science and medicine shaped and built the life they studied" (Cartwright 1995, xvii). However, while I agree with Cartwright and Stacey that cinematic technologies are the very means through which technologies of life emerge and I concur with Smelik that the scientific imaginary interrogates what it means to be human, natural, embodied and technological, I also want to suggest that a transplant imaginary evokes very specific ethical questions about migration, inequalities and postcolonial histories. Indeed, I would add that the transplant imaginary is concerned with the temporality of both the nation and the body. That is, a haunted time, where "what we normally exclude, or banish, or, more commonly, ... never even notice" (Gordon 2008, 24–25), is that which we are forced or compelled to engage with, to get close to and to perhaps remember in its partial or complete immateriality.[3]

The transplant imaginary as discussed in this article is connected to Lesley Sharp's work in *The Transplant Imaginary* insofar as the literary representations produce an economy of hope and are concerned with "questions about the boundaries of the human body, the importance of guarding its natal integrity, and what in fact qualifies as the 'natural'" (Sharp 2014, 43–44). Yet, unlike Sharp, I am not exploring transplantation or temporality as future-orientated, and thus the idea of the *imaginary* is less about what will or may come (Sharp's "what-if") and more about a significant and existing cultural phenomenon made manifest in literary and visual texts. It is thus about both the present and transplant's imagined connections to what might be viewed or understood as non-medical issues. It emphasizes an intimacy between organ transplantation and migration, violence, ethics, non-linear temporalities and intersubjective embodiments. My focus is Malika Mokeddem's (1998) *The Forbidden Woman* (originally published as *L'Interdite*) because of how it details migration as central to the transplant imaginary. It explicitly links colonial histories to contemporary biotechnological practices, and raises concerns around the relationality of national and individual self and other, which it maps onto a postcolonial politics of Algeria and France.[4]

I want to describe briefly the events that take place in the novel to give a sense of how the narrative of transplantation is interwoven with a history of post-independent Algeria. Mokeddem's *The Forbidden Woman* is set mainly in a small town, Aïn Nekhla, in Algeria. Aïn Nekhla is the birthplace of the main protagonist Sultana Medjahed who now works in Montpellier, France as a medical doctor. She returns to the town she left many years earlier because her friend and ex-lover Yacine Meziane has died. What unfolds is Sultana's fraught history with the local community in Aïn Nekhla, where when she was a young girl her father accidentally killed her mother and then left Sultana and her sister alone, resulting in the latter dying a few days later.

Ostracized because of her proximity to these deaths (Mokeddem 1998, 7), she subsequently takes refuge in the home of a white French doctor and his wife. Sultana recounts how she refused and in many ways was unable to conform to the changing institutional norms emerging after independence from the French colonial forces. *The Forbidden Woman* is haunted by the occupation of Algeria by France from 1848 through to 1962. It details the changing gender politics that emerged after the Algerian war of independence (1956–1962). Sultana's first-person narrative insists on a post-independence patriarchalization of Algerian society, where masculinity is instituted through an assertion of control over all public arenas and thus of apartheid-like gender relations.

The novel begins and ends with a chapter narrated by Sultana, and therefore her words frame the narrative of Vincent, the other protagonist, encouraging us to read his first-person narrative through her experience. Sultana's story alternates with chapters narrated by Vincent, who as a French, white, affluent man speaks of his recent kidney transplant. Vincent, a professor of mathematics at a prestigious Paris university, has taken a one-year sabbatical after both his near-death experience and his renewed sense of vitality. His words give space to both his uncertain sense of self and his intimacy with his female Algerian donor post-transplantation. Vincent needs to be close to his donor, but not by learning more about her as an individual. Rather, he is intent on exploring a sense of difference and otherness by visiting Algeria. *The Forbidden Woman* focuses on the meanings of racialized and sexed differences through Vincent's desire to understand what it means for him to have the kidney of an Algerian woman. To come close to the other and to feel altered by the other through the experience of organ transfer are presented through the problematics of race and sex structures in the context of post-independent Algeria and its continued neo-colonial relations with France.

Vincent's journey to Algeria, in order to understand his post-graft identity, mimics a colonial expedition where the search for the self takes place through an encounter with purported absolute difference. As Edward Said has eloquently demonstrated, the journey, in a colonial and oriental imaginary, constitutes the other through racial inferiority, national backwardness and atavistic imagery (Said 2003, 58). Yet, Vincent is the *postcolonial* tourist who uses economic power to undertake an existential journey where he hopes to find answers about the self in ever more "exotic" spaces. Jessica Jacobs argues that many tourists mimic the "famous colonial travellers", as they seek to "interact with the locals and 'understand' the culture" (Jacobs 2010, xiii). In other words, postcolonial spaces offer idyllic settings for the exploration of the European self, and therefore previously colonized nations re-emerge as sites of European interest, investment and epistemological appropriation. As Sultana tells Vincent: "And anyway, you know, desert freedom, escape, finding yourself … those are tourists' baggage. I have others" (Mokeddem 1998, 104). Vincent searches out difference in relation to the kidney donated by an Algerian woman by, first, visiting Parisian areas populated by North Africans and, second, by embarking on a journey to the donor's country of origin. Such facile definitions of difference point to how for the white, French man race is perceived as visible on the skin and through cultural practices (especially through food). However, such colonial assumptions are slowly undone as Mokeddem portrays the perfect tissue match for this white, French man as coming from the body of an Algerian woman. In other words, Mokeddem is using the biological to undo damaging colonial biological narratives. She turns to the visceral body not to argue that race is socially or culturally constructed, but to show the fallacy of the biology behind colonial science.

Vincent's journey is redolent of, without being equivalent to, such colonial and postcolonial journeys of searching out difference to constitute – and thus "find" – one's self. He is in search of a technologically altered self, which already feels of and close to this Algerian woman whose kidney could be said to live on inside him:

> She left me only the outline of her kidney, the feeling of her absence. I caressed her through this kidney. I tamed her in all the meanings of nothingness and to sail toward Algeria to the rhythm of the light autumn winds, to the rhythm of my blood travelling through her flesh, made me happy.
>
> (Mokeddem 1998, 22)

Vincent tries to control – "tame" – the woman who constitutes his sense of embodied self in a way that reflects his journey south as a colonial repetition. However, he can only feel "her absence", her continued elusiveness, which points to a different type of meeting between these two, a meeting where the white, French man does not have knowledge or control over the Algerian woman. Mokeddem evokes a potentially ethical encounter as she reaches to the concept of touch to imagine a coming together that is different from that of the French occupation of Algeria. Sara Ahmed suggests, "[T]ouch might allow us to challenge the very assumption that communication is about expression, or about transparency of meaning … Communication involves working with … 'that which fails to get across', … such that one ceases to inhabit the same place" (Ahmed 2000, 155–156). As Vincent insists, "She resisted me like the deeper meanings hidden under the superficial meanings of a word" (Mokeddem 1998, 22). He cannot control his donor and cannot define or have definitive knowledge of her. Indeed, his proximity is only possible through a touching of this other who, in her presence–absence, reminds us of this intimacy that remains unbridgeable and untranslatable. This limit of knowledge that is haunting him through the transplant scar suggests there is potential for co-existence in ways that do not mimic the logic of colonial occupation or of the postcolonial tourist. Such limits suggest a different type of encounter where Vincent's sense of self and world are destabilized and questioned, opening up a relationality between recipient and donor to an unimagined present intimacy haunted by unknowability.

Mokeddem brings together, in one body, a cultural history of assumed separation, hierarchical differences and continued oppression. That Vincent is able to undergo technologically advanced surgery, while those in Aïn Nekhla have access to very sparse medical facilities (ibid., 13), points not only to the unfair distribution of resources but also to how previously colonized bodies continue, in ever more innovative and disturbing ways, to maintain the lives of the ex-colonizers. On the one hand, the novel uses this biotechnological intervention to figure an alternative body politic where the colonial and postcolonial histories of France and Algeria are imagined through this sutured and scarred body. Here, the traces and what cannot be known haunt the body politic, calling attention to the absent and unarticulated histories of this scarred body. On the other hand, the novel is both an examination of how biotechnologies affect selfhood and an incisive critique of embodied and psychic violations caused by colonial rule and biotechnological interventions. Colonial damage to the self and to communal identity resonates with organ transplantation, and yet remains of a different order. Post-independence struggles for political, social and cultural viability and sustainability are compared with but distinguishable from the possible uncertainties of post-transplant selfhood. Indeed, the structure of the novel – where each chapter alternates between the names "Sultana" and "Vincent" – conveys how these histories and characters are intimately connected and yet that they cannot simply come together peacefully as if histories could be forgotten, as if those very histories do not continue to structure everyday life in Algeria and France. As the novel suggests, these histories might be intimately connected, in the way that an organ can be transplanted from one body to another. Yet, like organ transplantation, persistent interventions may be needed to ensure that the two (or the multiple) can live together in a state of constantly negotiated peace.

The transplant imaginary is thus to be conceived as this site of struggle where organ transplantation constitutes a world concerned with a selfhood that is not disembodied, bounded or separate. It is a spatialized imaginary transposed onto a colonial and postcolonial map where border anxieties expose how colonial inequalities continue to structure everyday life. This is how Ahmed defines postcoloniality:

> It is hence about the complexity between the present and the past, between the histories of European colonisation and contemporary forms of globalisation. That complexity cannot be reduced by either a notion that the present has broken from the past ... or that the present is simply continuous with the past.
>
> (Ahmed 2000, 11)

Postcoloniality is therefore temporally inflected in the way that Homi Bhabha (2004) and Gayatri Gopinath (2005) speak of the postcolonial nation. In other words, time is imagined as condensed, as a living of the past in the present because the past is not over, is not finished and may even need reworking or reconfiguring. Time is thus central to the transplant imaginary as the recipient lives the present through an attachment to an unknown time, a time of the donor that is present through the organ but absent in any cognizable form. Here, national time and biomedical time meet in their insistence on linear narratives of progression. What *The Forbidden Woman* insists upon is a time that is dissident from linear, forward progression, showing the continued haunting and sometimes necessary presence of the past in the present. If crossing the borders of time or an inability to keep time in order is part of the transplant imaginary, this is also because the bodily border has been cut in order to introduce the organ from an other into the self. In other words, linear time is of a self that is imagined as ordered, separate and bounded. Transplantation as a bodily crossing appeals to another time, a time that is both of the self and of the other. The transplant imaginary is simultaneously haunted by and evocative of postcolonial structures of violence and care, silenced histories, and the possibility of remembering the present absences.

Transplant temporalities and fleshy histories

Published autobiographical transplant stories are structured through a search for the origins of the recipient's transplanted organ. Claire Sylvia, a heart recipient, articulates this desire for knowledge: "And now, certain parts of [my] body – big, major, important parts – had been taken away and replaced with somebody else's. What did that *mean*? Who was this 'else'? And how did he, or it, fit into me?" (Sylvia 1997, 91). There is a need to understand who one is in relation to this donated body part or more specifically in relation to the deceased donor. In Sylvia's words: "I had always known who I was, but who was I *now*? I had been ripped in two and sewn back up, but something was different" (ibid., 91–92). Knowledge of the source of the organ frames the narrative as an explanation for any post-transplant changes in one's desires, tastes, body or needs (ibid., 90). The search for knowledge of the other is both a desire to know from where the organ that gives one a renewed sense of vitality originated and a need to know who one is now that the body and self have been altered.

Largely in contrast to transplant autobiographies, many postcolonial authors and scholars have been critical of nationalist narratives of origins, drawing out the reliance of such a politics on notions of so-called racial and sexual authenticity, normativity and purity (particularly for women).[5] *The Forbidden Woman* presents an ambiguous narrative of return, a return to a space that is both home and yet not home. Sultana states that it is a "return that isn't a return" (Mokeddem 1998, 67) and comments that being in Aïn Nekhla means that "I myself have become this exile, cut off from any attachment" (ibid., 66). She cannot return *home* because Aïn Nekhla rejected her as a young woman and continues to pose a violent threat to her existence. Familial national bonds are demystified as Sultana admits that any desire to return was cloaked in a "nostalgia" that was quickly "killed" on her arrival (ibid.). Mokeddem's refusal to write about *home* as an idyllic Algeria makes manifest both the continued precarity of women after independence and how migration may create multiple home spaces where one has a sense of not belonging anywhere (ibid., 112).

Yet if Mokeddem evokes familiar tropes of postcolonial literature and criticism, she imbibes this critique with Vincent's search for knowledge of his donor's previous national home life.[6] Where autobiographical narratives of transplantation stand somewhat in contrast to Mokeddem's resistance to the idea of returning to an idyllic origin, the novel's account of a kidney transplant critiques organ donation campaigns for rendering donor origins invisible:

> But I'd never thought of the "donor," and anyhow, who among us on the transplant waiting list concerns himself with the origin of the hoped-for organ? How can you think, or even imagine, that being part of this list automatically gives you the right to a kidney still walking around, if I may put it this way, still in the warmth of the original abdomen, still in the blood of its first body? … This kidney that I so yearned for belonged to no one, had no origin. It was born from the magic wand of a fairy named France Transplant.
>
> (ibid., 20)

While redolent of the anthropological work by Lesley Sharp (2006) and Renée Fox and Judith Swazey (1992), regarding how medical professionals constrain knowledge of the organ donor, the above critique does not stress the organ recipient's desire for access to information about the donor. Vincent wants to remember what came before his renewed vitality, to remember how someone had to live and die so that he could go on living. He uses gory fairy tale humour to point to the concealment of what has to happen during organ procurement. A fantasy narrative of origins is created to cover over the reality that those dying from organ failure are waiting for someone else to die in the hope that they will go on living. It is a refusal and/or inability to remember this haunting memory of another death. Mokeddem invites a reflection on whether by concealing origins we also silence histories of violence, violent deaths or, more simply, how organs travel between bodies. We may ask: is it only the recipient who is encouraged not to dwell on the possible unsavoury origins of donated organs, or is there a wider tolerance for not remembering that which disturbs stories of survival and continued life?

A national ontology is produced through a restructuring of time as national time. If the history of the nation is a forward-thrusting narrative, then the time of the nation is linear and teleological. Bhabha describes nationalist history as telling "the beads of sequential time like a rosary, seeking to establish serial, causal connections" (Bhabha 2004, 6). Sultana's return to an increasingly conservative post-independent Algeria makes manifest a political and national desire to restore a time that is prior to colonialism, a time that re-turns to an imagined pre-colonial and therefore authentic Algeria for the "real Algerian[s]" (Mokeddem 1998, 111). It seeks to purge this independent nation of its colonial relations with France. As Bhabha suggests, such nationalist sentiments and ideologies are constituted through a "forgetting to remember" that "totaliz[es] the people and unif[ies] the national will" (Bhabha 2004, 230). This is a wilful effort to restore that which never was, and that insists on certain markers of identity and specific (namely family) values to define such a time and to emphasize the only authentic way of being (in this case, Algerian). A post-independence ontology emerges through a pre-colonial time.

Similarly, one could argue that medical professionals want a static identity for transplant recipients, an originary identity and an authentic self to which the transplantee can return after transplantation. Sharp argues that the biomedical model of time "is wed to … a progression from diagnosis to treatment and cure" (Sharp 2006, 10). Both the nation and the hospital institute a sense of (national and individual) selfhood, which is bound and definable, to constitute an unchanging post-independence and post-transplant identity that are essentially prior to colonialism and transplantation. The "pre" is constitutive of the "post" and thus time moves forward only through a return to a pre-wounded self (wounded by colonialism and transplantation). This forgetting of Frenchness and returning to an authentic Algerian identity, along with this forgetting of the donor and returning to a self that already existed prior to transplantation, offer linear trajectories to a knowable national and individual self, which keep the normative structures of selfhood, time, the nation and biomedicine in place.

Many scholars have argued against such structures of time in experiences of illness and postcoloniality. Rita Charon (2006, 44) insists that "disease forecloses narrative coherence over time". Postcolonial time, according to Bhabha (2004, 220), "questions the teleological traditions of past and present". There is a convergence of postcolonial time and the temporality of narratives of illness. National and individual ontologies are thus not simply or only progressive, but rather constituted through the very ruptures of a past that will not remain confined to a time that could be (and often is) considered over and finished (namely the past). Describing how she feels to be back in the house that belonged to the French doctor and then to her ex-lover Yacine, Sultana states, "This house … in its grip, my memory panics between past and present. Time undergoes a contraction, a condensing" (Mokeddem 1998, 32). Sultana is not of the time of the nation; she has been unable to keep up with its linear narrative and its conservative values. She feels an "upheaval of present time" as if she is "losing [her] way between the past and the present" (ibid., 68). Sultana is experiencing the traumatic effects of loss and mourning, where memories merge with the present as if that person were still alive: "Last night I made love to Yacine" (ibid., 44). The traumatic loss of the man she has always loved confuses time and the boundary between self and other. As Judith Butler (2004, 23) suggests:

> What grief displays … is the thrall in which our relations with others hold us, in ways that we cannot always recount or explain, in ways that often

> interrupt the self-conscious account of ourselves as autonomous and in control.

Both Sultana's loss of Yacine and her traumatic experience of exile (of needing refuge from those around her and thus of "choosing" to leave) convey a living that is out of normative time and that undoes the nationalist need for a bounded, individualistic self. Mokeddem portrays time as contracted, as the past interrupts the present, as the self feels the impact of losing an other who is integral to the self. The return, which is not a return, brought about because of the death of an intimate one, instantiates loss as the undoing of the self and thus as an unravelling of time. She claims to have made love with Yacine and sees his presence, despite his death. Haunting, here, is a manifestation of Sultana's unwillingness and inability to let go of her dead friend. It is also a physical manifestation of her being out of time and place, and therefore her refusal to accept the current political climate of the post-independent nation.

Vincent is haunted by an absence that is present not only in the form of the scar, the physical trace, but also in what cannot be spoken: his near death experience and the death of an other. He describes his experience of organ transfer as follows:

> But in a city hospital, a piece of dead flesh calls you and waits for you in a cold receptacle. You will never be alone again. A dead kidney that is placed next to one of your own dead kidneys. … A dead kidney that lives again from your blood.
>
> (Mokeddem 1998, 91)

For Vincent, the time of death has already happened both in terms of his own dying body and the donor's deceased body. The time of life as linear and progressive is made possible only through the cessation of another life, and thus the time of life is interrupted through illness and death, restarted and yet no longer able to move only forward. Indeed, Vincent describes how he touches his scar to remember his donor: "My hand is on my kidney. My kidney beneath its scar. Its familiar curvature. Life fallen asleep, the presence–absence of my Siamese twin return to my memory" (ibid., 65). The repetition throughout the novel of the descriptor "presence–absence" and the invocation of the image of conjoined twins convey an inseparability of an alive (but previously dying) self from a (dead) other. Thus the present time is of a dead past that continues to live on in a second, warmer body: "my inner organs' suicide, my feeling of mutilation, my solitary past and present salutary state of being a twin, its strange solidarity" (ibid., 91). Like Nancy, Vincent describes strangeness as the encounter with his own body, his own sense of his "organs [refusing] to quietly do their work" (ibid., 90). His sense of death from within disturbs his self, disrupts his sense of continuity precisely because continued life is dependent on the death of an unknowable other. Death is not the past, this dead other is not absent, in the way that medical professionals might expect, but the donor is not present in any immanent way. Rather, she is simultaneously of death (i.e. absent) and of life, his life (i.e. present). Yet even the use of "his life" does not capture how Mokeddem describes transplantation as she reaches for the image of conjoined twins. While this is an image to which I will return in the following section, I want to suggest here that the repeated turn to the image of conjoined twins reinforces the inseparability of one person, space and time from another. The dead other is connected to the now revived Vincent and thus alive in the form of an organ and therefore connecting the past to the present and death to life. Transplant temporalities are haunted by histories that are silenced, just as national narratives are disrupted by women who refuse to forget the violence of post-independence politics.

Transplant and postcolonial temporalities are haunted by loss and grief. There is a literal haunting of the past in the present, where time may move forward (as it does in the novel) but always and only through the past in remembrance of silenced and unknowable histories. The transplant imaginary portrays the continuance of life and its inseparability from death, and therefore reveals a time different from the curative time of medicine and the progressive time of the nation. Here, time is interrupted, restarted and of the past without being determined by what was, and always living with what is and what may be.

Migration through difference, or organ transplantation

The Forbidden Woman portrays migration across national boundaries through a racialized biopolitics that deploys difference to render the migrant inferior (ibid., 112). Mokeddem's novel is redolent of Frantz Fanon's (1986) work on the racialized epidermal schema, which exposes how the skin is the experiential site through which colonial hierarchies are produced and consolidated. Mokeddem reaches to these familiar colonial tropes of the body as markers of difference to put into question a colonial scientific knowledge of racialized and sexed hierarchies. More specifically, she turns to biotechnologies and biology to undo the colonial structures of embodied difference. Furthermore, she destabilizes the security of the independent colonial subject who, in Hegelian terms, constitutes the other through his mastery, dominance and violence (Oliver 2001; McCormack 2014). Mokeddem, through transplantation, proposes an intersubjective relationality as constituting embodied existence to produce a subjectivity and selfhood not reliant on Hegel's structures of the slave and master dichotomy. Just as in Ahmed's ethics, where the self emerges through tactility, Vincent's post-transplant self comes into being as he touches his donor. He wants tactile intimacy with the one *already* touching him from the inside out. He wants to feel who she is, who they are together, as one and yet two:

> I catch myself caressing my transplant with a nostalgia of soul and fingertips, for this forever unknown body, this foreign woman with the

> same identity, my female Algerian twin. … I embrace her absence, I squeeze the emptiness of her presence. A kidney, almost nothing, a flaw, a simple twist of fate, unites us beyond life and death. We are a man and a woman, a Frenchman and an Algerian woman, Siamese twins, survival and death.
>
> (Mokeddem 1998, 21–22)

Margrit Shildrick (2002, 58) argues that "in western discourse, the evident privileging of singularity and autonomy implicitly premised on the bodily separation, and the value accorded bodily self-determination combine to erase any consideration that there might be other ways of being". Thus transplant rhetoric, with its emphasis on the separability of the organ donor from the organ recipient, instantiates ontology as distinct from and unaffected by embodiment (Sharp 2006; McCormack 2015). Ontological security is equivalent to bodily separation. Yet Vincent emphasizes their relationality through difference *and intimate togetherness.*

Conjoined twins, in the very way that Shildrick (2002) suggests in *Embodying the Monster*, provoke anxiety precisely because normative subjectivity is founded on oneness, the oneness of self in one body. Thus Mokeddem's turn to conjoined twins pronounces the experience of transplantation as out of the ordinary, and in so doing invites a reflection on how the self may be intimately connected to others. That is, transplantation shares a history, at least in the common imaginary, with that which disturbs ontological security and that which provokes anxieties about normative selfhood. Whereas conjoined twins are, as Shildrick demonstrates, often separated through surgery in an endeavour to create two separate and thus *normal* subjects (i.e. one person in one body), the description of transplantation suggests two bodies are being brought together in one person. In other words, the normative imperative to separate conjoined twins into singular bodies so as to cohere one self in one body is confounded in transplantation where two bodies are actively brought together, creating a sense of more than one in what may previously have been experienced as an individual self. Vincent is more than one, conjoined to an other through a kidney.

Vincent's sense of being with an other reaches to a universality that attempts to undo any notion of biological difference: "The mixed part inside me can't be seen, and I can't brandish my scars or my HLA [human leucocyte antigen] cartography to show my universality" (Mokeddem 1998, 52). Speaking about his donor as a perfect tissue match, he adds: "What a feeling to know that I had the same tissue identity as a woman and, moreover, a woman from elsewhere! Those who tell lies about the races would do well to take a glance at genetics!" (ibid., 91). He reaches to a notion of universality, redolent of the 1789 French Rights of Man, where all, except those who did not fit into the category of man, such as women and slaves, were considered equal. However, while French Republican universal values are the framework for an attempted destabilization of the connection between science, race and sex, the novel does not propose integration or assimilation as a response to how difference may co-exist. This is in stark contrast to contemporary French politics, which advocates "assimilation and the eradication of cultural difference" (Barclay 2011, xviii). Indeed, integration is undermined by a focus on transplantation, which shows how the assimilation of the other into the host body is not possible. That is, the other cannot become self; instead, the other's presence (especially in the form of the organ) continues to haunt the self, refusing to quietly labour away for the recipient solely on the latter's terms. Here, this biotechnological intervention proposes an ethics where the self does not remain intact. Rather, the self only becomes possible through its contact with an other, and the self is undone repeatedly by the other's visceral and haunting presences.

Fiona Barclay suggests that such a sense of haunted selfhood is apparent on a national level in France's continued neo-colonial relations:

> Specifically, the anxiety manifested in recent years with regard to the makeup of the nation and its identity, the relationship between the constituent parts of the body politic, and its guilt or otherwise at overlooked or forgotten episodes of its past would appear to testify to a nation haunted by the past from which it has sought to distance itself.
>
> (ibid., xxxiv)

I would therefore suggest that a transplant imaginary proposes an ethics where national and individual selfhood must be undone in its contact with others. As Ahmed suggests, "[The] ethical demand is that I must act about that which I cannot know, rather than act insofar as I know. I am moved by what does not belong to me" (Ahmed 2004, 31). Indeed, Vincent acts precisely because he can never know this other. He is moved by this present absence such that he can no longer inhabit that which may be conceived as a pre-transplant self. He is undone by that which he cannot know: the history of his donor. Furthermore, Vincent is uncertain whether he is integrating an other into his self or if he is being integrated into an other: "[The] donor opposed an insurmountable resistance, a stubbornness to remain another sensibility, a foreign particle, an anesthetized zone, thus erasing the recipient" (Mokeddem 1998, 117). Here, the donor is a significant presence, able to assert her being to the extent that she is able to take over an other. Living with difference, even when perfectly compatible, is a struggle, but Vincent comes to embody its potentiality with its "daily pills" (ibid., 118). The taking into the self of an other is figured less as a colonial conquest of the other, where one gains control of and knowledge over an other (be this through pharmaceuticals, bureaucracy or violence). Rather, it is an encounter where the other is the means through which the self may live or die. In other words, organ transfer shows how two supposedly different beings can live in one body. Yet, the need for pharmaceuticals, that one person is defined as dead and the unpredictability of continued life suggest a constant struggle where the white, French and male body lives on because the Algerian female body died for its survival. Here, the hauntings are of the dead donor *and* the unspoken histories of French colonial violence. How we can remember the silences and hear those who are silenced, and whether we can listen to these haunting absences, present only in their traces, is precisely what the transplant imaginary asks us to contemplate.

Haunting flesh, or living with the other

Jacques Derrida relates questions of justice and ethical responsibility to "those who *are not there*" and "to those who are no longer or who are not yet *present or living*" (Derrida 1994, xviii). He speaks of such present absences in terms of those subjected to state, national, colonial, racist and sexist violence (ibid.). A haunting absence draws attention to how that which is not there demands justice, by calling on an other to sense it and/or to remember it. Barclay argues, "[The] social invisibility of members of the community of immigrant origin within France means that, by virtue of their history ..., they function as embodied ghosts haunting the Hexagon" (Barclay 2011, xxxiv). Such present absences are taken up in Mokeddem's *The Forbidden Woman* to address the postcolonial body politic of Algeria and France. The transplanted body shows the scars of forgotten histories, specifically of how a deceased Algerian woman gave valuable viscera to a French man. The donor haunts Vincent to the extent that he feels intimate with her, as he feels her presence in what he understood previously as his own – distinct and discrete – body. Such a sense of two presences in *one* self raises questions about post-transplant ontology and our responsibility for others with whom we co-exist. Mokeddem is inviting a reflection on both the meaning of selfhood, particularly when body parts are moved from one supposed individual body to another, and how we may live with that which is structured and understood as different. Mokeddem's response to the colonial construction of hierarchical difference is to undermine its imagined scientific basis. She destabilizes the very biological narrative of colonialism, using biotechnologies to prove that sex and race are not biological markers of difference. Biotechnologies, for Mokeddem, give scientific veracity to the fact that organs and tissue may be compatible across those humans deemed definitively – and therefore biologically – different. She uses biology, in the form of tissue matching, to challenge the violence of a scientific epistemology based on derogatory cultural categories of hierarchical visual and physical differences.

The Forbidden Woman weaves together individual experiences of organ transplantation with post-independence histories of gender-based violence to bring forth a discussion of what it means to forget histories, especially racialized and sexed histories of care, occupation, health, violence and death. Asking Vincent about his organ transplant, Sultana wonders out loud whether there is a difference between him and her, "between the absence in one's self and the absence of one's self" (Mokeddem 1998, 86). These shared and yet different present absences index the loss of one's *own* kidneys; the absence and presence of the donor; the dispersal of one's self and the loss of home through migration; and the absence of one's narrative in colonial and post-independence histories. The novel does not simply fill these narrative gaps, although we do learn of Sultana's traumatic childhood and Vincent's transplant. Rather, the emphasis is placed on learning to live with these hauntings, and learning to understand what it means to live with the unknowable limits of the other and of history. This does not entail giving up on creating and imagining multiple histories. Rather, hauntings, present absences, demand our incessant attention, calling on us and often forcing us to engage with why they are unseeable, untouchable, and yet still there. By being absent and present they disturb our ontological, historical and biomedical certainties. We cannot therefore reach to those familiar methods of engaging with material others when trying to hear these immaterial or partially material others. Instead, we must seek out other ways to understand unnarrated, silenced or unspeakable events of colonial and intimate violence and organ donation. More specifically, we must address the consequences of silencing histories of embodied violence, exchange and colonization.

Mokeddem's text therefore evokes a transplant imaginary to convey an interrogation of how we may live with difference in a postcolonial and post-transplant context. The question of ethics is raised through a temporality that refutes the linear logic of national and healing time. Transplants and post-coloniality coincide through a haunting, a memory that will not go away and yet is not – and perhaps never can be – fully materialized. Sultana's history of segregation, migration, and racist and sexist violence draws out colonial and post-independent hierarchical structures that dominate both in and between Algeria and France. That her histories frame Vincent's narrative suggests his desire to understand his relationality to his donor is also a broader socio-political concern with the denigration and exclusion of difference. Mokeddem's turn to transplantation makes manifest an ethical openness to the other, captured through this imaginary of visceral exchange and intersubjective relationality. Organ transplantation renders apparent how the self emerges only through its indebtedness to others (in this case literally in the form of the donated organ). Yet, such openness is situated in histories of violence, reminding the reader how vulnerability may be simultaneously a space for ethical potentiality and of abuse. This vulnerability, Butler (2004) argues, is the potential to acknowledge and live with our intersubjective relationality, not by shoring up our defences, to protect what is perceived as an impermeable border, but by remaining open to that which makes life possible. In other words, by opening a space for recognition of self and other, interrelationality and France's indebtedness to and violence towards Algeria and its population, such an ethics is a way to imagine less violent postcolonial potentialities of being with others. Inter-subjective relationality is an openness that makes ontology possible, and in so doing demands a different (Butler would say non-violent) response. That is, a response-ability, which insists on remembering the national and individual relationship, and which is infinitely open to the other and in so being refutes the violent logic of the independent Hegelian subject.

A nationalist, in this case post-independent, body politic is produced through a cohesive, whole and unified selfhood, just as transplant teams insist that biotechnological interventions do not alter recipient identities. Yet, histories do not disappear, regardless of the labour put into trying to silence or deny them. Vincent wants to touch and get close to what he will never know, while also accepting that he can never gain total knowledge of his donor. Indeed, Vincent never seeks the details of his donor, but attempts to live another history by remembering who has had to die to maintain the metropolitan French body. This is a decolonizing act in its desire to remain with the haunting other, by not trying to appropriate the other, and by living with the constant undoing of the embodied self. Organ transplantation, as embodied by Vincent, requires a different response, where he lives with this other who is inside and outside – integral to and separate from – the self. In other words, he remembers the present absence. Similarly, Sultana demands a different type of engagement from both Algeria and France; she writes and speaks her histories of being subjected to violence, and makes apparent the rise of women-based political activism in Aïn Nekhla. Such an ethics of intersubjective relationality is a haunting, a repeated destabilization of the parameters of existing and accepted reality, especially as it is narrated through medical and national histories. Haunting gives a glimpse of spaces and times where the unspeakable, the silenced and the unspoken may break the teleologies of the familial nation and the need for Hegelian subjects. The transplant imaginary gives space and time to that which cannot and may never materialize, demanding we sense that which is there even when it is an immaterial presence, an invisible materiality or a haunting absence.

Notes

1 See p. 166 of *The Intruder* (Nancy 2008). Throughout this article, I will refer specifically to race and sex to evoke a production of categories that is built on and emerges from colonial ideologies and policies. It is the desire to engage with the meaning of the biological and what is at stake in such taxonomies that leads me to use both "sex" and "race". I am emphasizing the production of such categories and exploring how Mokeddem undermines them.

2 Mokeddem has multiple ways of referring to this "presence–absence", including "presence/absence" (Mokeddem 1998, 117) and "this absence transplanted into me" (ibid., 90).

3 A transplant imaginary may include multiple other factors, such as organ theft, unequal health care systems, futuristic consequences of organ donation, and so on. However, my point is that the figuring of transplantation as an issue of relationality and border crossing raises broader socio-political concerns that could be said to haunt the practice, experience and theories of transplantation, even when they may seem absent, unapparent or even unrelated. This does not mean that national concerns will always be at stake in all representations or experiences of transplantations.

4 It should be apparent that while my focus is Mokeddem's text, there are a multitude of texts that deal with a similar sense of a transplant imaginary. Indeed, I am arguing that such an imaginary is prominent in many cultural products.

5 See, for example, Gopinath (2005) and Niranjana (2006).
6 What is never mentioned in the novel is that the organ donor must have been living in France at the time of the donation and thus that her relation to Algeria is somewhat unclear, even if it is her place of birth.

References

Ahmed, S. 2000. *Strange Encounters: Embodied Others in Post-Coloniality*. London: Routledge.

Ahmed, S. 2004. *The Cultural Politics of Emotion*. Edinburgh: Edinburgh University Press.

Barclay, F. 2011. *Writing Postcolonial France: Haunting, Literature and the Maghreb*. Plymouth: Lexington Books.

Bhabha, H. 2004 [1994]. *The Location of Culture*. London: Routledge.

Butler, J. 2004. *Precarious Life: The Powers of Mourning and Violence*. London: Verso.

Cartwright, L. 1995. *Screening the Body: Tracing Medicine's Visual Culture*. Minneapolis: University of Minnesota Press.

Charon, R. 2006. *Narrative Medicine: Honoring the Stories of Illness*. Oxford and New York: Oxford University Press.

Derrida, J. 1994. *Specters of Marx*. Translated by Peggy Kamuf. New York: Routledge.

Fanon, F. 1986 [1952]. *Black Skin, White Masks*. Translated by Charles Lam Markmann, forewords by Ziauddin Sardar and Homi K. Bhabha. Sidmouth: Pluto Press.

Fox, R.C. and J.P. Swazey. 1992. *Spare Parts: Organ Replacement in American Society*. Oxford and New York: Oxford University Press.

Gopinath, G. 2005. *Impossible Desires: Queer Diasporas and South Asian Public Cultures*. Durham: Duke University Press.

Gordon, A. 2008 [1997]. *Ghostly Matters: Haunting and the Sociological Imaginations*. Minneapolis: University of Minnesota Press.

Jacobs, J. 2010. *Sex, Tourism and the Postcolonial Encounter*. Surrey: Ashgate.

McCormack, D. 2014. *Queer Postcolonial Narratives and the Ethics of Witnessing*. New York: Bloomsbury Academic Press.

McCormack, D. 2015. "Transplant Temporalities and Deadly Reproductive Futurity in Alejandro González Iñárritu's 21 Grams." *European Journal of Cultural Studies*. Prepublished May 29, DOI: 10.1177/1367549415585549.

Mokeddem, M. 1998. *The Forbidden Woman* (originally published as *L'Interdite*, 1993). Translated by K. Melissa Marcus. Lincoln: University of Nebraska Press.

Nancy, J.L. 2008. The Intruder. In: *Corpus*. Translated by Richard A. Rand. New York: Fordham University Press.

Niranjana, T. 2006. *Mobilizing India: Women, Music and Migration between India and Trinidad*. Durham: Duke University Press.

Oliver, K. 2001. *Witnessing: Beyond Recognition*. Minneapolis: University of Minnesota Press.

Said, E. 2003 [1978]. *Orientalism*. London: Penguin.

Sharp, L. 2006. *Strange Harvest: Organ Transplants, Denatured Bodies and the Transformed Self*. Berkeley: University of California Press.

Sharp, L. 2014. *The Transplant Imaginary: Mechanical Hearts, Animal Parts and Moral Thinking in Highly Experimental Science*. Berkeley: University of California Press.

Shildrick, S. 2002. *Embodying the Monster: Encounters with the Vulnerable Self.* London: Sage.

Smelik, A. 2010. *The Scientific Imaginary in Visual Culture.* Goettingen: V&R Unipress.

Stacey, J. 2010. *The Cinematic Life of the Gene.* Durham: Duke University Press.

Sylvia, C., with W. Novak. 1997. *A Change of Heart: The Extraordinary Story of a Man's Heart in a Woman's Body.* London: Little, Brown.

10 Managing hope and spiritual distress

The centrality of the doctor–patient relationship in combatting stem cell travel

Michael Humbracht, Insoo Hyun and Susanne Lundin

Introduction

Stem cell travel, commonly referred to as "stem cell tourism",[1] is a relatively new phenomenon that has garnered significant interest from a large field of actors. Stem cell travel refers to a form of medical mobility where patients from around the world travel to clinics for treatment with unproven commercial stem cell interventions for a wide variety of neurodegenerative diseases and debilitating disorders. Stem cell clinics employ a range of stem cell treatments that have not entered clinical trials or demonstrated efficacy, and that are often similar despite diseases or conditions having distinct aetiologies (Lau *et al.* 2008; Master *et al.* 2013). A majority of the debate about stem cell travel and how to conceptualize the issue has come via scholars who argue that the phenomenon needs to be combatted through strategies that target both supply and demand.

The most common approach for reducing supply is to strengthen regulatory frameworks that inhibit doctors (hereafter we refer to them as "purveyors") who treat patients with unproven stem cell therapies. While increased regulation has achieved some success, stem cell clinics have demonstrated an ability to resist regulation, revealing that creating global regulation of stem cell therapies is highly problematic and remains largely at the level of the political drawing board. To lessen demand, scholars and regulators have advocated informing both patients and doctors about stem cell therapies in general (Caplan and Levine 2010; Zarzeczny and Caulfield 2010; Master and Resnik 2011) and about clinics abroad. Although both approaches to combatting stem cell travel are important, they might not be enough. Elsewhere the second author argued that in order to truly reduce demand for stem cell travel, physicians have to be able to treat therapeutic hope and spiritual distress (Hyun 2013). In that article, however, therapeutic hope and spiritual distress were not developed in relation to the doctor–patient relationship; that is of critical importance if hope and spiritual distress are to be managed. There is a significant divide between how patients and physicians often frame and articulate stem cell travel with far-reaching consequences for combating the problem.

One patient with multiple sclerosis (MS) who went to Panama for stem cell treatments explained:

> I'm a huge stem cell supporter and advocate … There are so many that just want the hope and informed access to treatment that can help today, before permanent disability, incapacitation, and all hope is lost. Stem cells haven't cured my MS yet, but they gave me a second chance at continuing to fight my disease and be able to live another day!
>
> (MS patient, female, American)[2]

This very positive narrative on stem cell clinics differs from many physicians operating in Western contexts. A doctor who has worked extensively with stem cell research and Parkinson's disease explained his view regarding stem cell travel and purveyors carrying out treatments abroad:

> I think the main problem is that they [the clinics abroad] give the patients and relatives false hope and they lose a lot of money. And I think for the field of stem cell research the main the problem is that it destroys a lot, it creates some kind of feeling that stem cells do not work. Which I think is a very serious problem with stem cell tourism … I think it is unacceptable, but there are colleagues who don't have the moral stature.
>
> (Parkinson's disease physician and researcher, male, Swedish)[3]

The quotes here highlight the important and complex political economy that underpins stem cell travel: a political economy generated by doctors and patients, rooted in historical notions of healing and family care practice that are being reconfigured in modernity. Due to patient embeddedness in global bio-economies, patient-hood is no longer defined simply in hospitals and visiting rooms but also through a series of online networks and embodied experiences negotiated through travel routes. Connected, informed, reflexive and increasingly autonomous patients have brought the construction and mobilization of hope to new heights that subsequently raise important questions over responsibly for patient health and new complexities in patient agency. In parallel, doctors are increasingly required to maintain their role as family care providers while facing pressure to raise research funding in a competitive, commercialized and global landscape.

With this background, academic inquiry into changes in the doctor–patient relationship is central to combating stem cell travel. In this article, we aim to build on the discussion of managing therapeutic hope and spiritual distress (defined below) by examining the yet unexplored importance of the doctor–patient relationship as it pertains to patients seeking unproven commercial stem cell therapies. In addition, we argue that the notion of sharing[4] is of particular importance in conceptualizing both how patients construct notions of health and in defining potential avenues for improving the doctor–patient relationship. Or in other words, the ability of doctors and patients to share information, divergent notions of health and body, and embodied experiences play an important role in how doctors and patients build trust and negotiate ontological uncertainties.

To achieve this aim, we employ both a bioethical normative approach and the ethnological praxis approach. Ethnology is interested in how discourses, norms and values are "done" and "lived" in everyday life. It is then also possible to see how what one *should* do, the normative message, can be accepted by the person who receives the message, but she/he nevertheless often does quite differently in reality. That is, the message is often transformed according to her/his specific situation. With in-depth interviews and field observations it is possible to capture these contradictions and complex situations. The focus of this chapter is to combine knowledge of praxis with knowledge of normative perspectives and guidelines.

Patients and praxis

Understanding patient hope and the potential for strengthening trust are key to understanding the patient side of the doctor–patient relationship. Absent from research into stem cell travel is a complete understanding of the connections between patient hope and agency and how these connections have implications for patients' building or losing trust in medical authorities. While it may be tempting to view "hope" as a variant of wishful thinking, a mere passive longing for something good to happen, hope and agency are inextricably tied together for patients in the medical context. In the medical and psychological literature, therapeutic hope is defined as a patient's future health expectations that motivate him or her to take action. Patients who have therapeutic hope actively pursue perceived pathways toward disease amelioration or some other long-range personal goal for which disease amelioration is believed to be a stepping stone, such as familial independence or leading a meaningful life (Snyder 2000; Feudtner 2009; Hyun 2013). When a patient's active pursuit of these goals is thwarted – that is, when he or she loses therapeutic hope – the patient may slip into what some have termed "spiritual distress", understood as a lack of inner peace and purpose, and a general sense of loss of the meaningfulness of life (Ross 1995; Anandarajah and Hight 2001). Motivated by therapeutic hope, or the corollary, desire to stave off spiritual distress, patients may be tempted to actively pursue stem cell travel for their intractable medical conditions (Hyun 2013). This temptation can be exacerbated if patients also lose trust in medical authorities that discourage stem cell travel without providing meaningful alternative pathways to patients' ultimate goals, whatever they may be.

In addition, hope, patient agency and loss of trust are linked to shifting power relations between patients and medical authorities in late modernity. In stem cell travel, these changes are particularly evident with patients sharing information and experiences of treatments (both at home and abroad) through blogs, testimonials and online communities. As some of these online communities are created or explicitly supported by stem cell clinics (Chen and Gottweis 2011; Rachul 2011), many might question whether these testimonials are examples of "sharing" prompted by the stem cell clinics themselves to garner more business. On the other hand, however, others seem to suggest that many of these blogs are sincere attempts by patients to share their experiences (about how stem cell therapies affected their bodies) with what they may perceive as an "internet community" of similar patients in similar circumstances. One such community is www.stemcellpioneers.com, which claims to be entirely operated and moderated by patients, with no affiliation to physicians or stem cell clinics. The site has nearly two thousand members and aims to act as a platform for sharing information on a variety of different issues related to patient care, from current research on stem cells to regulation, and for sharing experiences between patients. One patient said this about a recent trip for stem cell therapy:

> So it has been 4 months since I received my stem cells. I actually ran the other day! Not long and not far, but I ran. I imagine it's what a baby feels like when it is learning to walk; that is, I could fall at any moment. But I still did it. Also, I am just about able to touch my toes again something I haven't been able to do in 3 years. I am also able to balance longer on one leg and go deeper in to my therapy stretches.[5]

When examining stories like this one shared between patients, it is important to understand not what hope *is*, but what hope make patients *do* (Frykman 2012). Hope is an affect grounded in the body, a physical reaction that defines a possible future on seemingly irrational grounds. Hope expresses something that we are *uncertain* about. The moment we know something for sure we are talking about confidence, which is slightly more cognitive and therefore less complicated. Thus, patient online communities affectively fuel hope and build a feeling of autonomy that drives efforts to help patients overcome obstacles, such as problems with funding trips and bureaucracy that might otherwise hinder stem cell travel (Chen and Gottweis 2011).

In addition, online communities exacerbate patient distrust and frustration with local or national healthcare systems and perceptions that healthcare and medical treatments are sluggish, lagging behind or bogged down by incumbent political authorities (Song 2010; Rachul 2011; Master *et al.* 2013). These perceptions are underpinned by a contemporary context where local doctors and medical institutions no longer have the hegemony over defining notions of health and body. Patient perceptions of health are generated from a baggage of experience, or praxis orientation, produced in and between several cultural contexts, which include doctors' examination rooms, virtual communities and clinics abroad. Patient perceptions are entangled with a contemporary paradigm of responsibility and consumption, but also with specific illness experiences, deeply and historically rooted patterns of thinking about healing and blogs, online communities, Facebook and other factors.

The medical gaze, as Foucault (1963) called it, is being subverted, or at least made more refractive by patients who are informed, connected and empowered and whose subjectivities are no longer defined only through local contexts (Prahalad and Ramaswamy 2004). Sharing in online communities is linked to growing dissatisfaction among patients with paternalistic doctor–patient relationships, and a desire to be more involved in their own healthcare decisions (Rachul 2011; Idvall *et al.* 2013). In our recent project *Therapies for the Future*,[6] investigating patient perceptions of their own involvement in medical care, patient autonomy was a common theme within the sample of patients:

> In meeting with the doctor, it's for me to have the space to be properly listened to and to have the possibility to speak up if I do not agree with the description of options or treatment of me as a patient.

Because patients are increasingly connected to circulating global flows of media, ideas and values on the body and health, patients are also increasingly obliged to re-imagine their locally situated notions of body and health (Appadurai 1996; Lock and Nguyen 2010). As a result, patients are also becoming more reflexive (Lash and Urry 1994) about their own health and how issues of health relate to their place in society, which increases patients' ability to take responsibility for and monitor their own health. Patient reflexivity between selves and medical structures is also leading to greater importance for transparency. Another patient online community that offers information on stem cells argues that, we "strive to be neutral when it comes to our own interests or that of any clinic or physician".[7] While the website's capacity for neutrality is highly ambiguous, what is clear from this statement and from patient online communities is a rise in patient desire for transparency in medical and health processes.

In addition, we argue patient autonomy should not be reduced to a heightened form of consumer capitalism. While patients may be consumers, at least in part, the increase in patient autonomy and responsibility for health is more complex and requires a more nuanced understanding. The academic literature on stem cell travel has mostly painted patients as consumers. This perception is limited as it hinges upon an assumption that globalization, and patients' embeddedness in global bio-economies, are synonymous with spreading neoliberalism. Furthermore, viewing patients simply as consumers reduces patients to passive subjects, does little to conceptualize patients as agents and is underpinned by a paternalistic framing that may inhibit the potential to combat stem cell travel.

The term stem cell "tourism", for example, is indicative of patients as consumers. "Tourism" is a highly problematic term that downplays the arduous and often painful experiences that many stem cell patients have described (Song 2010). The academic literature has superficially debated the term, mostly reducing the label of "tourism" to semantics. Instead, the term "tourism" is deeply reflective of how stem cell travel has been discursively embedded in many Western contexts. It matters that "tourism" has come to describe the phenomenon and not alternatives like "migration". Such a term would more reflect a failure of Western medicine to meet expectations for patient treatment, provide positive undertones to clinics abroad utilizing unproven therapies and emphasize the many difficulties patients face as they travel abroad to clinics. In this way, the term tourism is intimately linked to the political economy described in the introduction. The term tourism becomes morally loaded as it is connected to narratives created by physicians, medical authorities, academics and the media that frame patients as being "irrational" and easily susceptible consumers.[8]

This does not equate, however, to an understanding that patients cannot, or do not act as consumers. The packaging of stem cell trips, the use of advanced marketing techniques to potential stem cell patients (Petersen and Seear 2011) and the rise of stem cell treatments for non-debilitating diseases and injuries all point to patients creating notions of health through consumption, usually with the goading of purveyors eager to sell them their services. We need to recognize that patient hope and "irrational" logic result in part from their interconnectedness to global contexts and increases in market forces that together are putting strain on traditional notions of healing rooted in religious faith (Song 2010). As agents, patients involved in stem cell travel are capable, and indeed affectively compelled, to shape the world through a multitude of different roles such as consumers or pilgrims and alternate between roles in and between different contexts. Patient autonomy cannot simply be reduced to consumption or pilgrimage.

Patients are finding themselves placed in a multitude of cultural contexts that contribute to, or limit, hopes of gaining strength. Out of this complexity arises everything from hope to trust/distrust towards the healthcare system and trust/distrust towards "alternative" care systems. Complexity and uncertainty are essential to understanding patients as agents, and to understanding how to manage patient hope and build trust. Furthermore, patients should not be viewed as irrational but as expanding or reconfiguring patient rationality by attempting to cope with an increase in global flows such as electronic media and technology that interrogate historically rooted understandings of health and re-shape local contexts.

Doctors and praxis

Uncertainty and complexity are not reserved for patients; for physicians, notions of health and medical professionalism are also defined by tensions that have emerged in modernity. Traditionally, physicians have been guided in their profession by ethical norms which centre on a fiduciary responsibility to look after the best health interests of their patients and a broader social duty to use their expertise to benefit the health needs of the larger community. This combination of exclusive, institutionalized expertise and special societal obligations beyond the marketplace has been what sets the medical profession apart from other occupations. This traditional view of medical professionalism was recently reiterated in the Physician Charter, which was drafted by the American Board of Internal Medicine Foundation, the American College of Physicians Foundation–American Society of Internal Medicine, and the European Federation of Internal Medicine (ABIM Foundation *et al.* 2002; Munsie and Hyun 2014). The Physician Charter reaffirms the traditional ideal that physicians must place the interests of their patients above their own personal interests, including their own private financial interests. Market forces must not compromise the principle of the primacy of patient welfare. These traditional ideals of medical professionalism have started to erode in modern times, however, a fact that has motivated the drafting and wide dissemination of the Physician Charter (ABIM Foundation *et al.* 2002). Physicians today increasingly find themselves charged with generating research in a competitive and commercialized health environment. Against the ethos of the Physician Charter, medical professionals are now under constant pressure to move toward an institutionalized culture of commercialization that rewards innovation and technological development in a medical "marketplace". In the most egregious cases, purveyors of unproven stem cell treatments may try to justify their own self-interested commercial behaviour on these very grounds.

Following these broader trends, more mainstream stem cell researchers' and doctors' daily lives are in part constructed out of tensions between being situated in bio-economies while maintaining a conceptualization of patients and bodies as non-commercialized. To stay competitive, many reputable doctors and medical institutions follow a model of "flexible accumulation" that leverages their ability to impact scientific research by creating knowledge nodes that assemble scientific knowledge and technology in order to find new sources of value (Gottweis *et al.* 2009). This backdrop also sheds light on the hype about stem cell research that over the past decade has come from scientists, bioethicists and politicians who have enthusiastically portrayed its potential and contributed to the rise of stem cell travel. The reasons for this enthusiasm range from genuine idealism and optimism to practical realities for modern scientists who must simultaneously conduct rigorous research while also attracting industry and government funding by producing results that are clinically and commercially viable (Murdoch and Scott 2010). This situation is complicated even more by the fact that stem cell research is enormously controversial in many countries around the world. Due to ethical concerns, many nations have significantly limited the legal status of stem cell research and others have banned it all together (Mertes and Pennings 2008). The limits placed on doctors by their governments on ethical grounds places even more pressure on them to legitimate stem cell research.

Additionally, in order to conduct research physicians are increasingly required to secure bodies and human biological material. Bodies have become an important and valuable resource in transnational bio-economies (Idvall 2012) and are necessary to produce profitable research and therapies. In regard to stem cells, researchers and research institutions often strive to acquire intellectual property rights over stem cell lines. Researchers who have established patents in their stem cell lines have a strong commercial advantage because they can control the ways other researchers use their knowledge, and earn revenue through licensing and material transfer agreements (Gottweis *et al.* 2009). The US currently enjoys considerable advantage in stem cell patents (ibid.), while Europe recently banned stem cell patents, a move that was perceived by many as a blow to Europe's ability to be competitive in a global health market. Thus, a critical component of bio-economies is how physicians and research centres gain access to bodies and maintain control over materials, techniques and information.

As with patients, doctors as a professional category are no longer only defined locally but also through a synoptic gaze that has arisen through globalization (Bauman 1998), where medical professionals and authorities that once did the watching have also become the watched. Seen against this background, physicians' perceptions of patients as "irrational" or as being susceptible consumers can be explained in part as physicians acting out of historical notions of family care providers responsible for patient health, and in part as a discursive framing that condemns stem cell travel because of the danger it poses of delegitimizing stem cell research and therefore limiting physicians' ability to act in bio-economies.

Therefore, physician praxis arises from their embeddedness in overlapping and inter-articulating contexts of bio-economies, reflexive societies, research institutions and the private arena. As with patients, doctors constitute and are constituted by shifting between multiple roles in and between different contexts that are always culturally framed, and only one of which is interactions with patients. The discourse that has emerged from stem cell travel is in part the result of physicians attempting to uphold positions of power by defining what is correct knowledge and attempting to generate research funding (Lundin 2012). It would be fairer to say, however, that the internal professional logic and moral praxis that bind stem cell physicians is the result of attempting to make medical and research endeavours manageable, to create stability in an environment filled with personal and cultural insecurity (Lundin 2012; Bauman 1993).

The mobility politics of doctor–patient encounters

To combat stem cell travel, shared decision-making, responsibility and information are essential to building trust within the doctor–patient relationship. Thus, sharing is a critical concept for combatting stem cell travel.

To understand sharing and building trust, recognition is needed of how what is described above has both political and moral components. That is, stem cell travel is essentially a bio-politics (Foucault 2010) of mobility. Stem cell travel is generated, and resisted, through political economies where doctors and patients attempt to construct, conflate, deflate and disassemble dichotomies of hope and hype that embed or attempt to contain mobility within contexts of power. Importantly, these political economies morally ground the mobility of patients with either sedentary or mobile metaphysics that are known at the level of the body (Cresswell 2006). Thus, this is a politics where meaning is generated both discursively and through embodied practice. The point here is that the political economies that morally ground hope and hype play a significant role in generating or limiting the flows of patients. In addition, these politics are also a critical means through which to understand trust in the doctor–patient relationship and the role trust plays in stem cell travel.

Therefore, a key aspect of combatting stem cell travel is to understand how to strengthen the impact of the doctor–patient relationship within a context where the relationship is being de-centred from contemporary care. This could be achieved by considering how to *equally* increase the political and moral weight of doctor–patient interactions in relation to the variety of contexts that make up both doctor and patient lives. In order to better understand how this can be realized, we will present empirical material from the study that was mentioned above, *Therapies for the Future* – a study attempting to understand patient views on patient power and influence in healthcare. We do not intend to use patient perceptions as a prescription for creating a framework for doctor–patient relations; instead, we wish to use the empirical material to deepen our understanding of implicit tensions in doctor–patient relations, through the eyes of patients, in order to better inform our theoretical and ethical discussion of how to manage patient hope and spiritual distress.

A clear theme emerging from the interviews was a need for patient choice that should be well informed by interactive physicians and through an on-going dialogue. One patient explained, "it should be me that chooses and not the doctor, about what to do". Another patient went on to say that "doctors need to have more time for each patient to explain and have a working dialogue with the patient. It's really important if you are going to make things function".[9] In responding to questions posed by the researcher in an online discussion, many patients had clear ideas for what the basic components of this kind of functioning relationship should be. One patient wrote that there are three overall criteria essential to the relationship:

a) Transparency. It is important that the care process is transparent and that care language becomes understandable. The cause–consequence relationship must be made clear to educate patients.
b) Choices available. Without the option for choice (in the broad sense) patient power is meaningless.
c) Integrity. There is initially a clear power imbalance in the patient–physician relationship. If the doctor is too dominant, his power overrides part of the value of patient power.

Patients demonstrated a clear desire for more transparent and symmetrical relations. Patients did not, however, appear to feel that increased equality equates to full responsibility for their own care and they felt that receiving quality and effective medical treatment remains the top priority. It's not an all or nothing situation, there should be a lot more space than is probably available today for patients to speak up about their treatment and be able to choose between different alternatives, provided they are medically sound.

Increasing the role of patients in their own treatment does not mean a loss of importance for physicians or a decreased desire for quality care in patient lives. The study material reveals that while patients are inclined to play a larger role in treatment options, and to redraw borders of doctor–patient interaction, patients retain appreciation for the complexity of treatment and quality care. The patient who delineated the three criteria above for the doctor–patient relationship also wrote about how these criteria could work in practice:

a) Transparency. One way may well be like "My Account" which is increasingly being brought into the public sector, e.g. "My Medical Record", etc.
b) Choices available. Tricky. The aim of treatment is that to be healthy, which often are objective methods. Important choices do not make patient care anti-rational. A patient's emotional decision should not kidnap medical ethics.
c) Integrity. Here you have to build up clear rights–obligations in the patient-physician relationship.[10]

Patient reflexivity in relation to medical institutions, normative notions of health and paternalistic medical attitudes are reshaping patient socio-cultural outlooks towards self-monitoring extending patient reach in defining health. To combat stem cell travel an approach is needed that recognizes shifting power dynamics, rebuilds trust and yet remains effective in creating patient treatment options. Given the above, a paternalistic model will be unproductive and serve only to further erode the strength of the doctor–patient relationship. Considering that patients are aware that medical treatment is complex and that receiving sound medical care from qualified professionals remains important, the study material encourages the conclusion that an approach that incorporates patient self-monitoring and agency will better facilitate physicians' ability to impact decisions to go abroad for stem cell therapy.

We argue, therefore, that the doctor–patient relationship should be based on co-creating treatment as an experience (Prahalad and Ramaswamy 2004). The starting point for this approach, and for moving away from a paternalistic model, is to recognize that doctor–patient interactions are not communication situations where doctors advise patients to not become stem cell travellers but are encounters where people meet. Furthermore, these encounters are but one context, tied together with several other contexts and networks of interaction, for both doctors and patients, which together generate the political economies that encompass stem cell travel. In addition, co-creation implies recognition that patients are not "irrational". Instead, new patient logics are generated as a means of coping with uncertainty. This approach is entirely consistent with the bioethics normative and descriptive literature on the doctor–patient relationship, which traces its evolution over the past several decades from medical paternalism to much more mutually shared decision-making processes (Quill and Brody 1996; Brock 1993; Emanuel and Emanuel 1992). The ideal of shared medical decision-making between doctor and patient is offered as an ethically preferable alternative to paternalism, where the values and decision-making authority of the physician dominate, and to commercialism (the purveyors' favourite model), where the preferences and free choice of the "healthcare consumer" (that is, the patient) take precedence. Unlike decision-making in the marketplace, shared medical decision-making is appropriate for situations where uncertainty and therapeutic hope abound and alternative treatment choices impinge on different value systems of doctors and patients. The doctor–patient relationship as co-creation calls on doctors and patients to share decision-making power and openly acknowledge each other's limitations.

For doctors, the managing of hope and spiritual distress means building trust through the management of uncertainty. By presenting information and options, developing treatment with patients and learning about patients' experiences, physicians will be better able to encourage alternative actions, such as advising patients against going abroad for stem cell treatments. This is not to say that physicians are no longer responsible for patient health, or that they are no longer the main source of medical knowledge for patients, or that they are not responsible for building the environment in which the doctor–patient relationship takes place. This conceptualization does assume some transfer of responsibility to patients and that patients will play a larger role in the construction of treatment knowledge; the point, though, is that doctors and patients will both be better served by constructing and sharing responsibility and knowledge together more symmetrically. While this can mean that the doctor–patient relationship is more convoluted, it also means that the patients are more empowered and the relationship is more democratic.

Importantly, because patients understand and are involved, patients will be more willing to comply with the treatment modalities that they have jointly developed (Prahalad and Ramaswamy 2004). Critical to this process is transparency. A potential outcome for co-creating treatment options could be a doctor counselling a patient to not seek further treatment from unproven stem cell clinics but to invest her/his remaining time into the family. For doctors and patients to build the necessary trust to make such a suggestion possible, and for a patient to follow it, transparency on both sides is necessary. Physicians disclosing full information on treatments to patients are not enough. Doctors who share information and are reflexive and honest about issues facing contemporary physicians are better prepared for a transparent and non-paternalistic relationship with patients. In addition, part of that transparency includes the role patients, and their bodies, play in research centres acquiring resources. Resources that help build treatment options that solve a number of problems for various actors. Whether in regards to state-funded research projects that are underpinned by hopes that stem cells will lead to the extension of working life (Gottweis *et al.* 2009) or to research that can be patented and sold on a global scale by large companies, if trust is to be built between patients and physicians, patients need to be made aware of the role they and their bodies play in the ambitions of various organizations. While transparency may expose the quality of physician expertise (Prahalad and Ramaswamy 2004), and reveal to patients potentially contradictory interests doctors have as professionals, transparency on one side fosters transparency on the other and makes assessment of treatment options by patients easier.

It is here, in patient transparency, that doctors have the most significant potential to impact patient decisions about stem cell travel. First, patients who feel involved in treatment and who are willing to share intentions, thoughts and concerns about going abroad for stem cell treatments enable physicians to more directly engage with them about the risks of stem cell travel. Second, patients who have gone abroad for stem cell treatments and who are willing to share information about their experiences may be able to contribute to general knowledge about stem cells. In research contexts, it is clear that patients who volunteer for clinical trials share information about their bodies and the stem cell interventions applied therein for the sake of the greater good. In clinical care, it is clear that the patient is not involved in research. But in the case of innovative medical treatments (Lindvall and Hyun 2009) outside of clinical trials (e.g. stem cell travel) the role of the patient could be thought to be a bit wider, to include this element of "research participation" if best practice dictates that the treating clinician (with the patient's consent) ought to gather information that may be useful for initiating clinical trials. In this way, patients who seek out stem cell travel may have a role in sharing information about their bodies' responses to stem cell treatments (in an anonymous way of course) and also sharing their bodies, quite literally, with researchers who need to study how stem cells might impact the patients' conditions.

In addition, sharing information and transparency from purveyors is critical in maintaining the integrity of medical professionalism and trust within the doctor–patient relationship. The International Society for Stem Cell Research (ISSCR) and others have called for stem cell clinics to share information about the processes, types of patient cells and outcomes involved in their "therapies". This information has not been shared with other scientists and clinicians to date. The ISSCR guidelines state that after experience with a few patients, clinicians should try to gather information in order to help initiate a clinical trials process aimed at expanding generalizable knowledge. Ideally, the sharing of information should translate eventually into responsible bodily sharing through clinical investigation.

Conclusion

In sum, sharing is both fuel for stem cell travel, through patients sharing their cells with purveyors for profit and sharing personal information and experiences online, and also a means to combat stem cell travel, through doctors and patients sharing the construction of treatment and perhaps later through bodily sharing in the form of clinical research. To manage hope and spiritual distress, managing uncertainty is crucial. Managing uncertainty will serve to improve the ability to build trust within the doctor–patient relationship.[11] Trust is most likely to emerge in a doctor–patient relationship that co-creates treatment experiences together. This is largely a process of co-constituting professional and patient identity. In doing so, doctor–patient encounters are more strategically centred in political economies that attempt to control or produce patient mobility and that span and interconnect patient and physician praxis across several contexts. Furthermore, this does not assume the elimination of patient hope, but instead increases the potential to construct hope, or manage the uncertainty connected to patient praxis by doctors helping to direct hope in parallel with patients. Importantly, this conceptualization both recognizes and embraces the complexity of patient agency. The key resides in integrating the moral praxis of doctor–patient lives that underpins the political economies of stem cell travel. Importantly, co-creating treatment options is not the invention of some kind of new medical product but in fact resists commodification that often piggybacks on globalization. Here, we point out that products can be commoditized but experiences cannot (Prahalad and Ramaswamy 2004).

Acknowledgements

We would first of all like to thank Marsanna Petersen from our joint project *Therapies for the Future* for assisting with empirical data. We would also like to thank Olle Lindvall for sharing his knowledge of stem cell medicine and stem cell travel with us, and the participants at the workshop *Sharing Bodies within and across Borders*. Moreover, we wish to thank the editors of this book, Kristin Zeiler and Erik Malmqvist, for reading and commenting on an earlier version of this article. Susanne Lundin wrote her contribution during her stay as a fellow at Stellenbosch Institute for Advanced Study (STIAS), Wallenberg Research Centre at Stellenbosch University, Marais Street, Stellenbosch 7600, South Africa.

Notes

1 In this article we avoid understanding stem travel only through a lens of tourism because that has the adverse effect of discursively downplaying that patient trips abroad are also difficult, arduous and problem ridden (Song, 2010).
2 This quote was taken from a patient blog *I Love My New Stem Cells*, at www.ilovemynewstemcells.com. Accessed on January 17, 2014.
3 This quote was taken from an interview with a physician on March 13, 2013 as a part of the project *The Human Stem Cell: Health, Hope and Bio-economy*, coordinator S. Lundin, financed by The Swedish Foundation for Humanities and Social Sciences (see also Humbracht 2013).

4 The notion of sharing we are utilizing in this chapter is a form of social sharing. Somatic stem cells that are harvested from the patient's body are handled and circulated for a fee by other parties before being transferred back to the patient during the course of a commercial stem-cell-based treatment. In countries with very poor regulation of stem cell clinics, such as India and China, purveyors collect embryonic and foetal derived stem cells to transfer to their patients, a practice of bodily sharing in the more literal sense that is likely to grow unless more serious attempts at enforcing regulations are realized.

5 This quote was taken from www.stemcellpioneers.com, accessed on October 24, 2014. Individual patient information was not available.

6 *Therapies for the Future* is an interdisciplinary project financed by The Swedish Research Council, main coordinator Deniz Kirik, medical research, and principal investigator Susanne Lundin, cultural science. The empirical data presented here have been collected by ethnologist Marsanna Petersen. The authors would like to thank Marsanna Petersen for her important contribution to this article. Individual informant information is not available.

7 This quote was taken from www.patientsforstemcells.org, accessed on October 24, 2014.

8 Hence, in this chapter, we have employed the term stem cell travel to avoid reinforcing problematic connotations and political underpinnings linked to the term tourism.

9 These quotes were taken from two focus group studies within the project *Therapies for the Future*. Translations from Swedish to English were made by Michael Humbracht.

10 These quotes were taken from two focus group studies within the project *Therapies for the Future*. Translations from Swedish to English were made by Michael Humbracht.

11 Considering that this article argues for employing co-creation to reduce stem cell travel, it could be asserted that co-creation is simply a re-adapted form of paternalism that nevertheless attempts to protect patients from themselves and demonstrates little consideration for patient autonomy. We would, however, point out that the type of consumerism that underpins stem cell travel is also not the antidote to paternalism. Medical consumerism operates under an over-simplified and possibly pernicious conception of individual autonomy, where the exercise of autonomy translates into naked choice without the guidance of a medical professional. The notion of shared medical decision-making, which we have argued for here, operates under a more realistic and ethically responsible ideal of patient autonomy. We argue that because patient autonomy is guided through an interactive (and shared) process between physician and patient, patient autonomy is in fact respected. A more realistic approach to patient autonomy does not itself equate to paternalism. It is simply the better ethical conception of what autonomy requires.

References

ABIM Foundation (American Board of Internal Medicine Foundation), ACP–ASIM (American College of Physicians Foundation–American Society of Internal Medicine) and European Federation of Internal Medicine. 2002. "Medical Professionalism in the New Millennium: A Physician Charter." *Annals of Internal Medicine* 136(3): 520–522.

Anandarajah, G., and E. Hight. 2001. "Spirituality and Medical Practice: Using the HOPE Questions as a Practical Tool for Spiritual Assessment."*American Family Physician* 63(1): 81–88.

Appadurai, A. 1996. *Modernity at Large: Cultural Dimensions of Globalization*. Minneapolis, MN: University of Minnesota Press.

Bauman, Z. 1993. *Postmodern Ethics*. Malden, MA: Blackwell Publishing.

Bauman, Z. 1998. *Globalization: The Human Consequences*. Cambridge: Polity Press

Brock, D.W. 1993. "The Ideal of Shared Decision Making Between Physicians and Patients." In: *Life and Death: Philosophical Essays in Biomedical Ethics*, edited by D.W. Brock, 55–79. New York: Cambridge University Press.

Caplan, A., and B. Levine. 2010. "Hope, Hype and Help: Ethically Assessing the Growing Market in Stem Cell Therapies." *The American Journal of Bioethics* 10(5): 24–49.

Chen, H., and H. Gottweis. 2011. "Stem Cell Treatments in China: Rethinking the Patient Role in the Global Bio-Economy." *Bioethics* 27(4): 194–207.

Cresswell, T. 2006. *On the Move: Mobility in the Modern Western World*. New York: Routledge.

Emanuel, E., and L. Emanuel. L. 1992. "Four Models of the Physician–Patient Relationship." *JAMA* 267(16): 2221–2226.

Feudtner, C. 2009. "The Breadth of Hopes." *New England Journal of Medicine* 361(24): 2306–2307.

Foucault, M. 1963. *The Birth of the Clinic*. Paris: Presses Universitaires de France.

Foucault, M. 2010. *The Birth of Biopolitics: Lectures at the College De France 1978–79*. New York: Palgrave Macmillan.

Frykman, J. 2012. *Berörd: plats, kropp och ting i fenomemologisk kulturanalys*. Stockholm: Carlsson.

Gottweis, H., Salter, B., and C. Waldby. 2009. *The Global Politics of Human Embryonic Stem Cell Science: Regenerative Medicine in Transition*. New York: Palgrave Macmillan.

Humbracht, M. 2013. "State of the Art Report on Stem Cell Travel." Department of Arts and Cultural Sciences, Lund Unversity.

Hyun, I. 2013. "Therapeutic Hope, Spiritual Distress, and the Problem of Stem Cell Tourism." *Cell Stem Cell* 12(5): 505–507.

Idvall, M. 2012. "The Body as a Societal Resource in Transnational Giving: The Organ-Exchange Organizations of Scandiatransplant and Balttransplant." In: *The Body as a Gift, Resource, and Commodity: Exchanges Organs, Tissues and Cells in the 21st Century*, edited by M. Gunnarson and F. Svenaeus, 204–234. Huddinge: Södertörn University.

Idvall, M., Wiszmeg, A., and S. Lundin. 2013. "Focus Group Conversations on Clinical Possibilities and Risks within Parkinson Research: A Swedish Case Study." Department of Arts and Cultural Sciences, Lund University.

Lash, S., and J. Urry. 1994. *Economies of Signs and Space*. London: Sage Publications.

Lau, D., Ogbogu, U., Taylor, B., Stafinski, T., Menon, D., and T. Caulfield. 2008. "Stem Cell Clinics Online: The Direct-to-Consumer Portrayal of Stem Cell Medicine." *Cell Stem Cell*, 3(6): 591–594.

Lindvall, O., and I. Hyun. 2009. "Medical Innovation versus Stem Cell Tourism." *Science*, 324: 1664–1665.

Lock, M., and V.K. Nguyen. 2010. *An Anthropology of Biomedicine*. Chichester: Wiley-Blackwell Publications.

Lundin, S. 2012. "Moral Accounting. Ethics and Praxis in Biomedical Research." In: *The Atomized Body: The Cultural Life of Stem Cells, Genes and Neurons*, edited by M. Liljefors, S. Lundin and A. Wiszmeg, 13–39. Lund: Nordic Academic Press.

Master, Z., and D.B. Resnik. 2011. "Stem-cell Tourism and Scientific Responsibility." *EMBO Reports* 12(10): 992–995.

Master, Z., Zarzeczny, A., Rachul, C., and T. Caulfield. 2013. "What's Missing? Discussing Stem Cell Translational Research in Educational Information on Stem Cell 'Tourism'." *Journal of Law, Medicine and Ethics* 41(1): 254–268.

Mertes, H., and G.Pennings. 2008. "Embryonic Stem Cell-Derived Gametes and Genetic Parenthood: A Problematic Relationship." *Cambridge Quarterly of Healthcare Ethics* 17(1): 7–14.

Munsie, M., and I. Hyun. 2014. "A Question of Ethics: Selling Autologous Stem Cell Therapies Flaunts Professional Standards." *Stem Cell Research* 13(3): 647–653.

Murdoch, C.E., and C.T. Scott. 2010. "Stem Cell Tourism and the Power of Hope." *American Journal of Bioethics* 10(5): 16–23.

Petersen, A., and K. Seear. 2011. "Technologies of Hope: Techniques of the Online Advertising of Stem Cell Treatments." *New Genetics and Society* 30(4): 329–346.

Prahalad, C.K., and V. Ramaswamy. 2004. "Co-Creation Experiences: The Next Practice in Value Creation." *Journal of Interactive Marketing* 18(3): 5–14.

Quill, T.E., and H. Brody. 1996. "Physician Recommendations and Patient Autonomy: Finding a Balance between Physician Power and Patient Choice." *Annals of Internal Medicine* 125(9): 763–769.

Rachul, C. 2011. "'What Have I Got to Lose?': An Analysis of Stem Cell Therapy Patients' Blogs." *Health Law Review* 20(1): 5–8.

Ross, L. 1995. "The Spiritual Dimension: Its Importance to Patients' Health, Well Being and Quality of Life and Its Implication for Nursing Practice." *International Journal of Nursing Studies* 32(5): 457–468.

Snyder, C.R. 2000. "Hypothesis: There Is Hope." In: *Handbook of Hope: Theory, Measures, and Applications*, edited by C.R. Snyder, 3–21. San Diego: Academies Press.

Song, P. 2010. "Biotech Pilgrims and the Transnational Quest for Stem Cell Cures." *Medical Anthropology* 29(4): 384–402.

Zarzeczny, A., and T. Caulfield. 2010. "Stem Cell Tourism and Doctors' Duties to Minors – A View from Canada." *American Journal of Bioethics* 10(5): 3–15.

11 International clinical research and the problem of benefiting from injustice

Erik Malmqvist

Introduction: the case of Sam

Sam is a middle-aged, married father of two with stable employment, living in a Western European country. Sam has had asthma all his life, and in the last few years the symptoms have grown significantly worse. He experiences persistent chest tightness and shortness of breath, and is often fatigued due to lack of sleep. Several times he has suffered sudden and deeply distressing asthma attacks, which have forced him to seek emergency care. His multiple medications appear to provide increasingly little relief.

One day Sam's physician tells him that a new drug that might help him control his symptoms better has just appeared on the market, and suggests that he tries it. Sam eagerly follows the recommendation and is surprised by the result. He now breathes more easily and sleeps better, and he feels much more energized as a result. Also, the fear of a new attack, which used to cast gloom over his everyday existence, gradually retreats to the back of his mind. In all, Sam feels that the change of medications has greatly improved his quality of life.

About a year later, Sam comes across an in-depth newspaper article about his new drug. The article describes how the drug was developed through a series of clinical trials in India and other Asian countries. It is revealed that some of the subjects in the early-stage trials were desperately poor and chose to participate in pursuit of the modest financial reward. Some of the subjects in the late-stage trials were asthmatics who chose to participate because they had no other way of receiving treatment for their condition. Reading the story evokes strong moral discomfort in Sam. He is deeply concerned by the poverty and lack of access to healthcare among those who participated in the trials. What is especially disturbing, however, is the sense of being personally linked to these circumstances. Sam feels vaguely connected to the distant people on whom the drug was tested, as if the fact that he has benefited from the drug makes him in some sense responsible for their plight.

This chapter seeks to make sense of this sort of moral reaction. Does benefiting from the distant needy create any special responsibilities towards them? If so, why? These are very general questions for moral and political philosophy, of course, and they arise in many different contexts. However, my inquiry will focus specifically on the case of international clinical research. Such an inquiry potentially fills an important gap. The moral responsibilities of sponsors and investigators conducting research in developing countries are extensively discussed among bioethicists and codified in widely recognized ethical guidelines.[1] By contrast, the responsibilities (if any) of those who ultimately stand to benefit from much such research – patients in the developed world – remain unexamined.

To put my discussion into context I begin with a few remarks on international clinical research. I then specify the sort of responsibility that Sam's story illustrates, distinguishing it from other responsibilities. Thereafter I examine the view that benefiting from injustice (or wrongdoing) creates special responsibilities to the victims, arguing that the justifications that have been offered for such responsibilities fail to single out beneficiaries of Sam's kind. I end by exploring the idea that the responsibility to address structural injustice is a widely shared one.

On international clinical research

Sam's story is a fictional one, but it is by no means unrealistic. Clinical research is an increasingly global phenomenon. The number of clinical trials conducted in developing countries has risen dramatically over the last few decades. Although many trials are located in these countries in order to develop interventions aimed at their specific health problems, very often the conditions under study are primarily of concern for affluent countries. The intended consumers of the resulting drugs are commonly Western patients with chronic diseases like cancer, diabetes, cardiovascular disease and (as in Sam's case) asthma.

Different considerations motivate pharmaceutical firms and other sponsors to "offshore" their research to developing countries (Macklin 2004; Sunder Rajan 2007; Petryna 2009; Cooper and Waldby 2014). It is easier to find sufficient numbers of willing participants in these countries, and participants are generally on fewer drugs that may interact with the interventions under study. These factors allow trials to be completed more quickly and get clearer results, which is both scientifically and financially advantageous. Also, labour and service costs are much lower than in affluent countries. Another possible, more unseemly motive is sometimes suggested: the desire to sidestep the stringent regulations that affluent countries impose to protect research participants (Macklin 2004).

Developing countries themselves are often eager to host foreign research sponsors (Sunder Rajan 2007; Petryna 2009; Cooper and Waldby 2014). This is not surprising considering the substantial benefits that the research is thought to bring. Sponsors may need to invest considerably in improving the healthcare infrastructure and training personnel in host countries, and their activities often provide employment opportunities and stimulus to the local economy more generally. Moreover, foreign-sponsored trials may provide a rare chance for local patients to access state-of-the-art interventions or advanced medical expertise. In some countries trials run by the pharmaceutical industry appear to be increasingly counted on to provide the healthcare that a shrinking public sector can no longer offer (Petryna 2009).

Scholars and health advocacy groups have emphasized that participants in offshored research are often drawn from the poorest and most vulnerable. Typical participants in Phase 1 trials appear to be students, unemployed and contingent labourers trying to supplement their income, while those who enrol in Phase 2 and 3 trials are commonly patients seeking treatments that they cannot otherwise afford or access (Sunder Rajan 2007; Petryna 2009; Wemos 2010; Cooper and Waldby 2014). This reliance on the poor and medically under-served is no doubt part of the reason why concerns about exploitation loom large in bioethical debates about international clinical research (Macklin 2004; Hawkins and Emanuel 2008).

Distinguishing responsibilities

Let us return to the responsibility that Sam feels he has towards those on whom his drug was tested. My inquiry into this sense of responsibility might be challenged in two different ways, and these challenges need to be addressed for the purpose of a clearer discussion. First, it might be argued that there is little point in trying to understand Sam's felt responsibility, because it is clearly groundless. Surely it is not his fault that people in India are poor and lack access to healthcare. Their hardships are not due to any wrongdoing on his part. However, we must distinguish between two senses of the term "responsibility". An agent may be responsible for some harm in the sense of being morally to blame for its occurrence or in the sense of being morally required to address it.[2] One sort of responsibility need not entail the other, and what is at issue here is the latter. More precisely, I shall be concerned with what David Miller calls a "remedial responsibility", a term he defines as follows:

> To be remedially responsible for a bad situation means to have a special responsibility to put the bad situation right, in other words to be picked out, either individually or along with others, as having a responsibility towards the deprived or suffering party that is not shared equally among all agents.
>
> (Miller 2001, 454)

The second objection is that we need not consider individuals like Sam to find out who is remedially responsible for the plight of those who participated in the trials of his drug, because there are other more plausible candidates. Many believe that the responsibility to alleviate poverty and ill health in developing countries primarily lies with these countries' own governments. Others believe that it lies, in large part at least, with the governments of affluent countries, or with international bodies such as the World Health Organization (WHO) and the World Trade Organization (WTO) (Pogge 2008). It has also been argued that pharmaceutical companies have a special responsibility to meet the health needs of the global poor (Resnik 2001).

Whatever the merits of these different views on responsibility for poverty and ill health, however, none of them precludes attributing responsibility to individuals like Sam. Holding one agent responsible for addressing some harm does not relieve others of responsibility in that regard. Consider a trivial example: if a child makes a mess at a party, both parents can clearly be responsible for cleaning up and apologizing to the hosts. Of course, the precise relationship between their respective responsibilities can be debated. The point here is simply that the fact that one is responsible does not absolve the other. Analogously, Sam may well be remedially responsible for poverty and ill health in India even if other agents also have such responsibilities.

Sam's sense of being responsible for the situation in India by virtue of having benefited from it cannot, then, be dismissed by pointing towards the responsibilities of other agents. Nor does it seem reducible to whatever responsibility he himself may have for that situation *qua* citizen or consumer or fellow human being. It may be that Sam, as a citizen of a democratic state, has an obligation to support political representatives willing to ameliorate the situation. Or, to the extent that the situation arises from structural processes that Sam participates in as a consumer in a global economy, it may be that he ought to contribute to changing these processes (Young 2011). Or it may be that Sam has a general humanitarian duty to assist the desperately needy, wherever they are, if he can do so at little personal cost (Singer 1972).

All these responsibilities may be attributed to Sam as an individual. However, none of them seems *specific* enough to match the sense of responsibility awoken in him upon learning about the development of his medication. The first is shared equally with all voters in Sam's country, the second is shared with other consumers in a global economy, and the third seems (in principle at least) to be shared with all fellow moral agents. None weighs more (or less) heavily on Sam than on other members of these groups. Nor are they responsibilities directed specifically towards the needy in India – from whom Sam has benefited – but rather towards the needy in general.

The special responsibility that Sam senses he has, if it exists, is not only distinct from the more familiar responsibilities that he or other agents may have. Also, its *basis* appears to be different. Following Miller (2001), it is commonly thought that an agent may be remedially responsible for a bad situation because of her causal or moral responsibility for that situation's occurrence, her communal ties to those suffering from it, or her capacity to alleviate it. Remedial responsibilities for poverty and ill health in developing countries tend to be assigned on precisely these grounds (Barry and Raworth 2002). For instance, those inclined to hold foreign states responsible often appeal to the role of these states in creating these problems in the first place (moral or causal responsibility) (Pogge 2008). Those who instead assign these responsibilities to local governments emphasize the special relationship between members of political or cultural communities and the special duties of mutual aid that such ties create (community). And proponents of an individual duty to aid stress how easy it is for relatively affluent individuals to bring great relief through modest financial donations (capacity) (Singer 1972).

None of these familiar bases of responsibility seem to single out Sam. He surely has no special ties to the needy in India; it is difficult to think of anyone more aptly described as strangers to him. Nor has he played any special role in bringing about their difficult circumstances. And although he certainly has some capacity to help remedy these circumstances by contributing to humanitarian organizations, for instance, he is no more so capable than anyone else equally well off.

The only thing that relates Sam, specifically, to the needy in India, specifically, appears to be the fact that he has *benefited* from them. And so we need to ask whether benefiting from other people's hardships, in and of itself, could give rise to an obligation to help remedy these hardships.

Benefiting from injustice

Several philosophers have recently argued that agents may acquire remedial responsibilities for bad situations in a way that Miller's account does not recognize, namely, by benefiting from such situations. More specifically, they have argued that *benefiting from injustice* (or wrongdoing) may give rise to responsibilities towards its victims (Gosseries 2004; Anwander 2005, 2009; Pogge 2005, 2008; Butt 2007, 2014; Goodin and Barry 2014). This is thought to be the case even when the beneficiaries were not involved in committing the injustice from which they benefit, and even absent any special tie to the victims or special capacity to put their situation right. Different versions of this view have been advanced to attribute special responsibilities to the beneficiaries of human-induced climate change (Gosseries 2004), global poverty (Anwander 2005, 2008; Pogge 2005, 2008) and historic injustices such as slavery (Butt 2007). Can the sort of responsibility that Sam feels he has in our case be accounted for along similar lines?

Two distinct questions need to be addressed here. First, is Sam a beneficiary of injustice? Second, if he is, does he therefore carry a remedial responsibility towards its victims?

As to the first question, Sam has no doubt benefited from changing medications. He is better off than he was on his old drug, and better off than he would have been had he remained on that drug. But does this gain count as benefiting *from an injustice*? There are two senses in which it might. First, it may be that one or more of the trials needed to bring the new drug to market were wrongfully carried out, for instance because the participants were coerced, exploited or exposed to excessive risk. Sam would then be the beneficiary of wrongdoing on the part of the sponsors or researchers. Second, it may be that the background situation of the participants, their poverty and lack of access to healthcare, is unjust, and that Sam has benefited from this situation because it facilitated the development of the drug. Sam would then be the beneficiary of a structural injustice rather than some individual wrongful act.[3]

I will set aside benefiting from injustice in the first sense. If the sponsors or researchers wronged the participants, surely *they* should put things right, not Sam. Perhaps Sam would still have some responsibility to put pressure on them (or even to "take up the slack") should they fail to act. But his responsibility *qua* beneficiary of wrongdoing would then be derived from their duty *qua* wrongdoers. Our inquiry into benefiting as a basis for remedial responsibility would require a detour over moral responsibility as a basis for remedial responsibility, which would take us too far afield. We are likely to get a clearer picture of beneficiaries' responsibilities in cases where these are not derivative of more stringent primary duties of wrongdoers. Let us therefore assume, for the purposes of this chapter, that the sponsors or researchers did nothing wrong when carrying out the research.[4]

Sam may still have benefited from injustice in the second sense. Indeed, it seems highly likely that he has. We should, I believe, regard the circumstances of the trial participants – their poverty and lack of access to healthcare – as unjust rather than merely unfortunate. This claim is admittedly not indisputable. How much economic security and healthcare individuals are entitled to is a subject of deep disagreement among theorists of domestic and global justice. Nor is it an especially controversial claim, however. Most theorists agree, albeit for different reasons, that access to at least a minimum level of these key goods ought to be provided as a matter of justice (Millum 2012). From this perspective, poverty, when avoidable and severe enough, and avoidable lack of access to essential drugs and basic healthcare, are indeed unjust rather than merely unfortunate. Of course, it remains open for debate what constitutes a minimum level and consequently who falls below it. But poor Indians enrolling in clinical trials to make a living or to obtain asthma treatment they need but cannot afford or access seem like strong candidates.

Not only should we regard the circumstances of the trial participants as unjust. There is also, I believe, reason to think that Sam has benefited from these unjust circumstances. He appears to be better off than he would have been under just circumstances – i.e. if the participants were not unjustly poor and had adequate access to care. In other words, his gain appears to be counterfactually dependent on their unjust situation.[5] If participants were less poor and had better access to care they would surely have been less eager to enrol in the trials. The financial reward would have been less effective in attracting healthy volunteers to the early-phase trials. And asthma patients would have been much less likely to enrol in later-phase trials in pursuit of needed but unavailable treatments. It seems highly likely that participant recruitment would have been more complicated, and that the entire trial process would have been slower in consequence. And so the new drug would have become available to patients in developed countries later, if at all.[6]

Benefiting as a basis for responsibility

It seems, then, that Sam is indeed a beneficiary of injustice. This brings us to the second question raised above: is he therefore remedially responsible for that injustice? Let us look at some justifications that have been offered for attributing remedial responsibilities to innocent beneficiaries of injustice.

Restitution

One way of benefiting from injustice is by coming to possess some good that was wrongly taken from someone else. One then normally has a duty to return the good to its rightful owner. For example, if somebody steals your bike, gives it to me and then disappears without a trace, then surely I am required to return the bike to you. You have a claim in restitution to the bike, and it would be wrong for me to keep it. In many cases, the responsibilities of innocent beneficiaries of injustice can be accounted for along these lines. For instance, recipients of the spoils of colonialism should clearly return what was taken even if they were not originally involved in the plunder (Anwander 2005, 42).

However, other cases of benefiting from injustice do not seem to involve receiving any misappropriated good. Whatever responsibility the beneficiaries may then have cannot be grounded in the victims' claim in restitution (Anwander 2009, 181). In the case of Sam, for instance, no tangible item has been wrongly taken from sick and poor Indians and transferred to him. His responsibility to them, if any, cannot be construed in terms of returning what is rightly theirs.

Benefiting at the victim's expense

Some appeal to intuitively plausible cases to justify remedial responsibilities on the part of beneficiaries of injustice. Robert E. Goodin and Christian Barry discuss a case where you were admitted to Harvard only because your father had bribed an admissions officer. Thanks to your Harvard education you have led a much happier and more successful life than you otherwise would have. You learn about your father's misdeed after his death many years later: "clearing up his estate, you find all the correspondence, along with the cancelled check" (Goodin and Barry 2014, 365). You also learn who was the next candidate on the Harvard waitlist for your year and was therefore denied admission because of what your father did. Tracking this person down, "you discover he was distraught at not getting into Harvard, became an auto mechanic instead, had been in and out of gaol, and led a pretty unhappy life quite generally in consequence of not being admitted to Harvard" (ibid.).

In this case, Goodin and Barry contend, you must compensate the victim of your father's misdeed. You should relinquish (some or all of) the benefits received as a result of your wrongful admission to cover (some or all of) the loss he suffered as a result of not getting into Harvard.

Daniel Butt (2007) offers a more fanciful but structurally similar case. A, B, C and D possess a quarter each of the land on a remote island. They are entirely self-sufficient and are strangers to each other. Only one crop will grow on the island, and each person must produce 200 kilos of it annually to support herself. Hard-working A produces 700 kilos the first year, whereas laid-back B, C and D only produce 200 kilos each. The next year, D tries to boost her crop by diverting water from B's and C's land to her own. But the plan misfires: the water is instead diverted away from C's land and her own and onto B's land. Consequently, C and D have no crop to harvest, whereas B surprisingly is able to harvest 400 kilos. A is unaffected by these events and harvests 700 kilos again. Destitute, D kills herself in despair. C will also surely die unless A or B give her the needed 200 kilos.

Who should come to C's assistance? Butt (2007, 132–133) notes that among Miller's grounds for distributing remedial responsibilities, only capacity applies; neither A nor B are causally or morally responsible for C's situation, and neither has any communal ties to C. A has more crop to spare than B and is therefore more capable of offering assistance. However, Butt suggests, it intuitively seems more appropriate that B helps C. After all, B has directly profited from the heinous act that left C destitute.

In both these cases it does seem intuitively plausible that the beneficiary of injustice should come to the victim's assistance. What drives this intuition, I suspect, is the fact that the beneficiary gains at the victim's expense. You took the other candidate's place in the Harvard class. And, in the island case, the same water that would have allowed C to produce the needed 200 kilos instead allows B to produce an extra 200 kilos. There is a direct relationship between the beneficiary's gain and the victim's loss. What one has gained, the other has lost.

In cases where the relationship between gains and losses is more attenuated, the claim that the beneficiary should assist the victim seems to lose some of its intuitive plausibility. Suppose in the Harvard case that the unsuccessful candidate turns out to be an unusually skilled auto mechanic, but has too low self-esteem to charge more than the going rate for his services. Then it would seem that his customers have benefited from an injustice. Had your father not bribed the admissions officer, the candidate would have been admitted to Harvard, and would not be performing excellent but underpriced car repairs. Yet it seems strange to require the customers to compensate the candidate for what he has lost in consequence of being denied admission. Their benefit seems too incidental to his loss.

Turning now to the case under discussion, does Sam benefit *at the expense of* the sick and poor in India? It would appear that he does not. His gain does not directly correspond to any loss for anyone among them. They are equally sick and poor regardless of whether he receives the drug or not. Sam is not like the candidate who was wrongly given the talented auto mechanic's place at Harvard, but rather more like the customers who benefit from the mechanic's underpriced services. He benefits from an injustice, to be sure, but not at the expense of its victims.

Sam's case is, then, importantly disanalogous with cases of the sort advanced to support the view that benefiting from injustice or wrongdoing creates remedial responsibilities towards its victims. Thus, we cannot appeal to the intuitive force of such cases to establish that patients in affluent countries are responsible for correcting the unjust conditions wherein their drugs are developed. Nor can we appeal to them to justify remedial responsibilities in other situations where the relationship between gains and losses is similarly attenuated, as is arguably often true of benefiting from structural injustices more generally.

Consistency

Butt appeals to consistency to explain why beneficiaries of injustice have special duties to the victims. He claims that "taking our nature as moral agents seriously requires not only that we be willing not to commit acts of injustice ourselves, but that we hold a genuine aversion to injustice and its lasting effects" (Butt 2007, 143). To condemn an act as unjust, but to refuse to reverse or mitigate its effects because one has benefited from it is to make "a conceptual error", he says: "The refusal undermines the condemnation" (ibid.).

In a later paper, Butt restates this claim as follows:

> there is an inconsistency in our moral outlook if we condemn actions which harm others as wrong, and so maintain that they should not have taken place, but then refuse to perform actions within our power which would make the actual world closer to a world where the wrongdoing did not occur.
>
> (Butt 2014, 340)

Perhaps there is indeed something inconsistent about refusing to rectify a situation that one sincerely holds to be unjust. But such refusal seems equally inconsistent regardless of whether one has benefited from that situation or not. If genuine moral agency requires aversion to injustice, including a commitment to reversing or mitigating its effects, then that is presumably true of all moral agents. So if successful, Butt's argument establishes a general responsibility to rectify injustices, not a special responsibility on the part of their beneficiaries.

Free-riding

Some invoke the notion of free-riding to justify remedial responsibilities on the part of innocent beneficiaries of injustice (Gosseries 2004; Anwander 2009). Generally speaking, a free-rider is someone who "obtains a benefit without paying all or part of its cost" (Gauthier 1986, 96). Though usually considered unfair when it comes to enjoying public goods without bearing some share of the cost of their provision (e.g. tax evasion, using public transportation without a ticket), free-riding in this generic sense is not always wrong. We do not usually criticize children or gift recipients for failing to "pay" for the benefits received from parents or donors. Thus, if the concept of free-riding is to do real moral work, such as justifying remedial responsibilities, it seems to require some qualification.

Norbert Anwander advances a more specific concept – *moral* free-riding – to explain why the costs of alleviating global poverty should partially be shouldered by those who benefit from that situation. He writes:

> Moral free-riding … occurs when someone profits from another person's wrongful action, from situations of injustice, or generally from what is morally unacceptable, without covering some appropriate share of the moral costs … The moral costs of an unjust global order are whatever it takes to reform it and alleviate the misery it has caused. Since morally there should be no injustice and no severe poverty, you are a moral free-rider if you benefit from such an order, while not sharing in the task of making it morally acceptable. You let others bear the costs of the morally necessary task of eradicating global poverty while profiting from its causes.
>
> (Anwander 2009, 185–186)

This approach appears better suited than an unqualified appeal to free-riding to justify the sort of responsibility under discussion. Sam has not just received a free benefit; what he has benefited from is, after all, a morally unacceptable situation. Those who work to improve that situation without benefiting from it might, not unreasonably, find it unfair that they should carry that burden alone, while beneficiaries like Sam refuse to join their efforts (ibid., 186).

But is there really anything *special* about innocent beneficiaries of injustice in this respect? Anwander (plausibly) assumes that eradicating global poverty is a collective moral task, shared among some group of agents. When somebody benefits from global poverty she becomes a member of that group. If she then fails to contribute to the task she free-rides on those who do contribute. However, it seems that we could say something similar about other group members who fail to contribute. They benefit in the sense that they shift a cost they otherwise would bear onto others. They too are free-riders, unfairly benefiting from other people's efforts.

Anticipating this critique, Anwander (ibid., 187–188) grants that anyone who ought to contribute to some collective moral task but fails to do so free-rides on the contributors. However, he argues, this form of free-riding differs from *moral* free-riding because it presupposes a duty to contribute. Moral free-riders, by contrast, need not have any such pre-existing duty. The concept of moral free-riding explains how agents can *acquire* the duty to contribute in the first place: by benefiting from a situation that morally ought not to be.

But if this is indeed a difference it seems to dissolve with the passing of time. Suppose at time *t* that agent A has no duty to contribute to the collective effort of remedying some unacceptable situation S. At t^1, A benefits from S, thus acquiring the duty to do her fair share in that effort. Suppose then that at t^2, A still hasn't done any remedying. Presumably A is now a free-rider in precisely the same sense as anyone else who fails to bear their share of the collective burden. She benefits from having her share borne by others.

Perhaps considerations of free-riding can explain how innocent beneficiaries of injustice can acquire remedial responsibilities. More importantly, however, such considerations point towards a more general ethical concern. *Anyone* who should help remedying injustice – regardless of how they acquired that responsibility – but fails to do so, free-rides on the efforts of others. Their moral shortcoming is ultimately the same as that of unhelpful beneficiaries. In other words, considerations of free-riding do not seem to *single out* those who, like Sam, innocently benefit from injustice.

Shared responsibility

We have examined four different justifications for attributing special responsibilities for remedying injustice to those who benefit from it. The former two failed to explain how such responsibilities can arise in cases like Sam's, where the benefits are not akin to stolen goods and do not come at the victim's expense. The latter two did provide some basis for assigning responsibility to beneficiaries even in such cases, but only by invoking considerations that are by no means unique to them. To the extent that they should be moved by these considerations to help remedying injustice, so too should many others.

Our failure to find a compelling justification for singling out beneficiaries of structural injustices as remedially responsible for these injustices might inspire two different sorts of response. First, one might take this failure as a challenge to find a better justification. The intuition that there is something morally special about Sam might seem sufficiently strong to warrant further inquiry. The question is what might explain it. Second, one might abandon the search for such a justification and instead, in keeping with my last remarks in the preceding paragraph, embrace something like what Iris Marion Young (2011) calls political responsibility. In Young's view, the task of remediating structural injustice should not be assigned to any particular agent at the exclusion of others. Rather, it is a task we must *all* engage in through collective action.

Although these are different responses, I suspect that their implications might ultimately be similar. Even if a compelling reason for fixing special responsibilities on beneficiaries of injustice is found, it is unclear that this will allow us to pick out any very limited set of responsible agents. I have focused on the case of Sam because it illustrates the phenomenon of benefiting from injustice especially vividly. But is Sam really all that different from most of us citizens of affluent countries? It is not unlikely that the low prices and high living standard we enjoy are to a large extent contingent on conditions that should be labelled unjust. Would these advantages be as great if workers in poor countries were able to secure decent wages and working conditions, for instance, or if their governments were not unfairly disadvantaged in international trade negotiations? These are admittedly complex questions, but it does not seem at all implausible that they should ultimately be answered in the negative, i.e. that most or all of us are indeed beneficiaries of injustice.[7] Thus, even if benefiting from injustice creates special responsibilities, such responsibilities may well be very widespread.

Suppose these reflections are on the right track: the responsibility to address structural injustice is in fact one that all or most of us share. Is Sam's sense of being especially responsible then entirely misguided? Not necessarily. To see why, it is important to note that emphasizing our shared responsibility is an incomplete response to structural injustice. To say that everyone is responsible for correcting a problem is, in a way, to say that nobody has any *special* responsibility in this regard. And then there is a clear risk that the problem will remain unaddressed (cf. Miller 2001, 469). Thus, even a model of shared responsibility requires some conception of how the sharing involved is supposed to occur. Everyone should presumably do *something*, but not the *same* thing, nor carry an equal portion of the collective burden. So the problem of distributing responsibilities remains, albeit in a modified form.

Here the considerations captured in Miller's four principles – causal responsibility, moral responsibility, capacity and community – all seem relevant. How closely connected an agent is to the victims of injustice in these four ways will help determine the appropriate shape and size of her contribution to the shared task of remediating their situation. This brings us back once more to the main topic of this chapter. Does benefiting from structural injustice – or rather, if most or all are beneficiaries, benefiting more than others – also affect one's responsibility to engage in the collective endeavour to rectify it? Should one do more than others? Young thinks so: "Persons and institutions that are relatively privileged within structural processes have greater responsibilities than others to take actions to undermine injustice" (Young 2011, 145). I shall end by exploring that idea a little further. Receiving benefits from structural injustice can, I think, make a difference to an agent's pre-existing responsibility to address that injustice – although what ultimately matters is not benefiting from injustice as such.

One way in which benefiting makes a difference is simple. To benefit is by definition to be made better off in some respect. There are at least two reasons why this might plausibly be thought to affect the extent to which one is responsible to address injustice. First, in the case of all material (e.g. money) and many non-material benefits (e.g. time), one will, very crudely put, have more "resources" to spare than one otherwise would. In Miller's terms, one's capacity to provide remedy increases, and so does one's remedial responsibility. Second, regardless of the type of benefit, the better off should arguably carry a larger portion of shared burdens than the worse off, other things being equal. A broadly egalitarian concern for distributive fairness seems to demand as much. To concretize these rather abstract points, consider the case of Sam again. It is reasonable to think that Sam should shoulder a larger portion of the shared task of rectifying structural injustice after changing medications than before. This is both because he simply *can* do more – he is no longer plagued by fatigue and fear of a new attack – and because fairness requires that he relieve other, less advantaged participants in that endeavour of some of their burdens.

Note that what carries the weight here are considerations of capacity and fairness, not benefiting from injustice per se. These considerations require anyone – beneficiary of injustice or not – who is better off than Sam to do more than he, other things being equal. Note also that these considerations are silent as to where remedial efforts should be directed. Sam has an increased responsibility to help remediate injustice in general, not (necessarily) an increased responsibility to the sick and poor Indians from whom he has benefited.

Another way that benefiting can make a difference is by undermining one common defence for failing to shoulder one's responsibility. In today's interconnected and mediatized world, ignorance of the situation of the sick and poor abroad is an increasingly poor excuse for withholding assistance. We generally know, or could and should know, that help is needed. The ignorance excuse can be further weakened by the receipt of benefits from that situation. In many cases, beneficiaries of injustice should be mindful of the provenance of their gains. For instance, it is reasonable to expect consumers of cheap apparel to ask themselves how it is possible for prices to be so low. Pursuing that thought further, they may well conclude that current prices are made possible by exploitative working conditions in manufacturing countries or more generally by the harsh structural circumstances that make working under such conditions seem attractive. And ignorance is then no tenable excuse for failing to help improve these circumstances. Unlike the considerations of capacity and fairness examined above, this one does affect agents' responsibilities to address the specific injustices they have benefited from, not only their duty to promote justice in general. Among all the harms one could help repair, it makes sense to target those one is most acutely aware of.

Of course, in Sam's case it is the newspaper story rather than the receipt of the drug that calls attention to the situation of the Indian trial participants. But perhaps Sam's thoughts should have been drawn in that direction already when he was presented with the drug. The role of international research in developing new pharmaceuticals is increasingly publicly known, and the great disparities in power and wealth that constitute the backdrop of that research are no secret. In any case, even if ignorance remains credible before reading the story it certainly does not thereafter.

The upshot of these rather sketchy remarks is this. There appears to be some substance to Sam's sense of being especially responsible for the sick and poor Indians from whom he has benefited. This is because he is better placed to provide assistance than before changing medications and because he can no longer credibly ignore their plight, not because he has benefited from injustice per se. More importantly, however, this sort of responsibility should be much more widely felt. Perhaps we find Sam's case striking not because his position is unusual, but because we do not sufficiently acknowledge being similarly positioned.

Acknowledgements

I wish to thank audiences at Linköping University and participants in the symposium *Sharing Bodies within and across Borders* for stimulating discussions of earlier versions of this chapter. Special thanks to Joe Millum for his insightful comments.

Notes

1 For a selection of the bioethical literature on this issue, see Emanuel *et al.* (2004), Macklin (2004), Hawkins and Emanuel (2008). The most influential set of ethical guidelines pertaining to international research is found in the Declaration of Helsinki (WMA 2013).
2 The distinction between blame-based, "backward-looking" and non-blame-based, "forward-looking" conceptions of responsibility has been noted by a number of philosophers. See, in particular, Jonas (1984) and Young (2011). Although these are distinct conceptions, they are nonetheless related. First, if an agent is morally required to address some harm but fails to do so, she will arguably eventually be to blame for that harm's persistence (Nussbaum 2011, xxi). Second, as discussed below, blameworthiness for the occurrence of some harm is one among several reasons why an agent may be required to address that harm.
3 On the distinction between structural injustice and individual wrongdoing, see Young (2011).
4 It must be stressed that this is a methodological assumption. It may well be that many trials in developing countries are in fact wrongfully carried out. Indeed, I am inclined to think that this is not uncommonly the case (Malmqvist 2015). However, in such cases sponsors or researchers should make amends, and the responsibilities of innocent beneficiaries of the research are of secondary importance at best. To better focus on these latter responsibilities we should therefore bracket any wrongdoing on the sponsors' or researchers' part.
5 Two remarks on the notion of benefiting employed here. First, I assume that in this context the baseline against which benefits are to be measured is a counterfactual (rather than a temporal or moral) one. Roughly, this means that P benefits from X if P is better off than P would have been had X not occurred or obtained (rather than being better off than before X occurred/obtained or better off than P ought to be). Second, because benefiting simply means to be made better off it does not require that one acts. Benefiting from injustice should thus be distinguished from *taking advantage* of injustice in the active sense of using somebody else's unjust position to advance one's own ends. Such advantage-taking raises a different set of ethical issues (Malmqvist 2013). For an essentially identical account of what it means to benefit from injustice, see Anwander (2009, 181–182).
6 For detailed analyses of the importance of poverty and lack of access to healthcare for participant recruitment and ultimately for successful pharmaceutical research, see Sunder Rajan (2007) and Cooper and Waldby (2014).
7 For compelling arguments to this effect, see Pogge (2008). While Pogge emphasizes the role of governments of affluent countries in perpetuating global injustice, he also points out that these governments act in the interest of their citizens.

References

Anwander, N. 2005. "Contributing and Benefiting: Two Grounds for Duties to the Victims of Injustice." *Ethics and International Affairs* 19: 39–45.

Anwander, N. 2009. "World Poverty and Moral Free-Riding: The Obligations of Those Who Profit from Global Injustice." In: *Absolute Poverty and Global Justice: Empirical Data, Moral Theories, Initiatives*, edited by E. Mack, N. Schramm and S. Klasen, 179–189. Farnham: Ashgate.

Barry, C., and K. Raworth. 2002. "Access to Medicines and the Rhetoric of Responsibility." *Ethics and International Affairs* 16(2): 57–70.

Butt, D. 2007. "On Benefiting from Injustice." *Canadian Journal of Philosophy* 37: 129–152.

Butt, D. 2014. "'A Doctrine Quite New and Altogether Untenable': Defending the Beneficiary Pays Principle." *Journal of Applied Philosophy* 31: 336–348.

Cooper, M., and C. Waldby. 2014. *Clinical Labor: Tissue Donors and Research Subjects in the Global Bioeconomy.* Durham: Duke University Press.

Emanuel, E.J., Wendler, D., Killen, J., and C. Grady. 2004. "What Makes Clinical Research in Developing Countries Ethical? The Benchmarks of Ethical Research." *Journal of Infectious Diseases* 189: 930–937.

Gauthier, D. 1986. *Morals by Agreement.* Oxford: Clarendon Press.

Goodin, R.E., and C. Barry 2014. "Benefiting from the Wrong-Doing of Others." *Journal of Applied Philosophy* 31: 363–376.

Gosseries, A. 2004. "Historical Emissions and Free-Riding." *Ethical Perspectives* 11(1): 36–60.

Hawkins, J., and E.J. Emanuel, eds. 2008. *Exploitation and Developing Countries: The Ethics of Clinical Research.* Princeton: Princeton University Press.

Jonas, H. 1984. *The Imperative of Responsibility. In Search of an Ethics for the Technological Age.* Chicago: University of Chicago Press.

Macklin, R. 2004. *Double Standards in Medical Research in Developing Countries.* Cambridge: Cambridge University Press.

Malmqvist, E. 2013. "Taking Advantage of Injustice." *Social Theory and Practice* 39: 557–580.

Malmqvist, E. 2015. "Better to Exploit than to Neglect? International Clinical Research and the Non-Worseness Claim." *Journal of Applied Philosophy.* Prepublished August 10, DOI: 10.1111/japp.12153.

Miller, D. 2001. "Distributing Responsibilities." *Journal of Political Philosophy* 9: 453–471.

Millum, J. 2012. "Global Bioethics and Political Theory." In: *Global Justice and Bioethics*, edited by J. Millum and E.J. Emanuel, 17–42. New York: Oxford University Press.

Nussbaum, M. 2011. "Foreword." In: Young, I.M. *Responsibility for Justice*, ix–xxv. Oxford: Oxford University Press.

Petryna, A. 2009. *When Experiments Travel: Clinical Trials and the Global Search for Human Subjects.* Princeton: Princeton University Press.

Pogge, T. 2005. "Severe Poverty as a Violation of Negative Duties." *Ethics and International Affairs* 19: 55–83.

Pogge, T. 2008. *World Poverty and Human Rights*, 2nd ed. Cambridge: Polity Press.

Resnik, D.B. 2001. "Developing Drugs for the Developing World: An Economic, Legal, Moral, and Political Dilemma." *Developing World Bioethics* 1(1): 11–32.

Singer, P. 1972. "Famine, Affluence, and Morality." *Philosophy and Public Affairs* 1: 229–243.

Sunder Rajan, K. 2007. "Experimental Values: Indian Clinical Trials and Surplus Health." *New Left Review* 45: 67–88.

Wemos. 2010. *The Globalization of Clinical Trials: Testimonies from Human Subjects.* Amsterdam: Wemos Foundation.

WMA (World Medical Association). 2013. "World Medical Association Declaration of Helsinki: Ethical Principles for Medical Research Involving Human Subjects." *Journal of the American Medical Association*, 310: 2191–2194.

Young, I.M. 2011. *Responsibility for Justice.* Oxford: Oxford University Press.

12 The ethics of transactions in an unjust world

Joseph Millum

Introduction

The world is indisputably unjust and will remain so for the foreseeable future. No individual has the power to correct this injustice. For the vast majority of people, even if they do everything they can, the corrective change they will produce will be small. Individual agents must therefore interact with one another against a backdrop of injustice.

Individual transactions across national borders or between citizens of different states are increasingly common. These include straightforward trade in goods, but also trans-national hiring, medical tourism, international collaborative medical research, the sharing of biological samples and other uses of people's bodies. With these transactions, even in cases where all parties agree to arrangements that are expected to benefit all, there may be concerns about ethical violations. For example, in 2007, Indonesia stopped sharing H5N1 (avian flu) samples with the World Health Organization's Global Influenza Surveillance Network because it judged that its population was highly unlikely to get access to a vaccine in the event of a flu pandemic (Sedyaningsih *et al.* 2008). There have been multiple cases in which complaints have been raised about the uncompensated or under-compensated use of indigenous people's knowledge about their environment (Millum 2010). One of the central debates in international research ethics concerns the distribution of benefits and burdens when research is conducted in low- and middle-income countries (LMICs). It is widely believed that in order for such research to be ethical, benefits must accrue not just to research participants, but to the populations from which those participants are drawn (Emanuel 2008).

In this chapter I examine the ethics of benefit-sharing agreements between victims and beneficiaries of injustice in the context of trans-national bodily giving, selling and sharing.[1] Some obligations are the same no matter who the parties to a transaction are. Prohibitions on threats, fraud and harm apply universally and their application to transactions in unjust contexts is not disputed. I identify three sources of obligations that are affected by unjust background conditions. First, power disparities may illegitimately influence transactions in unintentional ways. Second, better-off individuals have duties to ameliorate injustices. These are not specifically duties to those with whom they interact, though often it is easier and more effective to help those with whom one already interacts. Third, the power differentials created by injustice make exploitative transactions more likely. I summarize a transactional account of exploitation and argue that avoiding exploitation is usually easiest to achieve by ensuring that the more powerful party does not obtain an unfair share of the benefits from the transaction. The beneficiaries of a transaction do not have to be only those individuals directly involved in it. Indeed, in many cases it is thought that exploitation may be avoided by providing benefits to third parties. Working out when this is the case requires working out when a contribution or burden on another's behalf can count towards the avoidance of exploitation. I argue that it counts as such in two main cases: when the people in question are already involved in relationships of reciprocation, and when the individual making the contribution identifies with the interests of the other people.

The central examples I draw on in this chapter concern trans-national forms of exchange involving people's bodies. However, my conclusions apply equally to individuals transacting in any unjust institutional context, including within a single nation-state. I also mostly discuss the responsibilities of individual actors. However, this should not be taken to refer to just single, isolated people. Any entity that acts as one may count here, including corporations, ministries of health, families and so on.

Background injustice

In claiming that the world is unjust I am making a claim about *distributive* justice. That is, I am making a claim about the way that institutions, broadly construed, distribute rights, duties and – most importantly for the cases I am interested in – resources.[2] These institutions include national governments, but also trans-national institutions, such as the United Nations and the World Trade Organization. The fact that there are institutions that greatly affect the distribution of resources internationally implies that the international order can be appraised to see if it is just. More or less all political philosophers – from cosmopolitans to statists – agree that there are principles of justice that apply globally.[3] The fact that more than three billion people live on less than US$2.50 a day, while the 500 richest people are worth approximately US$3.5 trillion is powerful evidence that the global order is in fact unjust (Shah 2013). I do not argue further for this claim here.

The transactions that generate particular ethical concern as a result of this injustice are those that take place between parties who are in different positions in the global order. We may be concerned, for example, when pharmaceutical companies transact with marginalized indigenous communities, or when rich high-income-country patients with kidney failure transact with very poor potential organ donors. Paradigmatically, then, we are concerned about interactions between two parties, in which some sort of exchange is proposed, from which one or both parties stand to benefit, and in which the parties start from very unequal positions.[4] In general, we are also naturally more concerned with the wrongs that may be committed by the more powerful party, though, of course, all parties will have obligations.[5]

Wrongs can be committed within such transactions as a result of how the terms of the transaction – what is to be done and how the costs and benefits of doing so are to be distributed – are reached. For example, one person might get her way by presenting a credible threat to the other party and thereby coercing him. She might engage in deception about what benefits will accrue to him and thereby fraudulently set the terms. Or she might act negligently while doing what they agreed to and unjustifiably harm him. Both parties may have difficulty communicating and agreeing on mutually acceptable terms simply because of cultural, linguistic, or other impediments to a straightforward interaction. But all of these are problems that frequently arise independent of whether the actors involved are beneficiaries or victims of injustice. Although they require careful ethical analysis, they do not require it because of injustice.

Three ethical concerns may arise as a result of background injustice. First, when powerful actors interact with those who have little power, even if they do not use unethical means to influence the terms of a transaction, they may be perceived as doing so. For example, a doctor may not be threatening her patients when she asks them to participate in a clinical trial in which she is involved. However, a patient may have no other access to care, and may not feel empowered to insist on his rights; he may perceive a threat of abandonment, even if one does not exist. Such possibilities entail *pro tanto* duties on the parties to a transaction to make reasonable efforts to ensure that the transaction not only does not wrong people, but is not perceived as doing so. I do not think this is controversial. The real challenges in this regard do not require ethical analysis but are practical problems concerning how to fulfil this obligation in different cultural and socio-economic contexts. Second, those who are the beneficiaries of injustice, those who are more powerful and those who have more resources, may have greater duties to ameliorate injustice. It might be thought that these duties are owed to those with whom they transact. I consider this possibility in the next section. Finally, transactions can be fully consensual and mutually beneficial, and yet be exploitative. The power differentials created by injustice make exploitative transactions more likely. I examine at length how exploitation can be avoided in the latter part of the chapter.

The obligation to redress injustice

The area of transitional theory that addresses the obligations of individuals to work towards justice is underdeveloped. However, it is plausible that moral agents who live under unjust social institutions have some obligations to make those institutions more just, especially if they are the beneficiaries of injustice.

It is also possible that outsiders to unjust social institutions have some, perhaps weaker, obligations to improve them. These obligations may be both negative – requiring non-interference with others who are working towards justice – and positive – requiring that the agent perform actions in order to improve her social institutions. They are likely to be *pro tanto* obligations, that is, obligations that can be outweighed by countervailing obligations and limited in how much they can demand of individual agents.

In order to work out whether such obligations affect the ethics of transactions, it is necessary to consider what grounds them. There are two plausible candidates. First, they might be grounded in a general duty of beneficence, such as the duty of rescue.[6] If this is correct, then there will be no additional duties that arise in virtue of interacting with the victims of injustice: duties of beneficence arise because of the extent of the needs of the beneficiary and the ability of the benefactor to provide a benefit, not because of any interaction between them. However, it may be that it is easier to provide benefits to people with whom one interacts. For example, a duty like the duty to rescue is more likely to be triggered when interacting with people who are likely to need rescuing. The fact that benefactor and (potential) victim are already interacting can dramatically lower the cost to the benefactor of providing the rescue. If a researcher collecting blood samples from a population is already screening them for HIV, the cost of contacting HIV-positive donors and referring them to a clinic is likely to be low. Such referral could therefore be an ethically required rescue. By contrast, there is not a rescue-based obligation to engage with such a population in the first place to ensure that those who are HIV-positive are identified and referred.[7]

Second, one may acquire duties in virtue of being part of an unjust system. In order to avoid complicity with injustice it might be necessary to do something to repair the injustice, even if you did not create it yourself (Malmqvist 2013). Someone who is the beneficiary of injustice, such as someone who receives more than her fair share of the gains of social cooperation, might have an obligation on the basis of restitution to help repair the system. Again, a prior interaction might make such repair or restitution easier. For example, a high-income-country scientist is better placed to upgrade the infrastructure and train technicians at a research site in a low-income country when she is actually collaborating with that site. Again, however, the duty would not be related to any interactions between the beneficiaries and victims of injustice. Such duties would stand even if they were otherwise isolated from one another.

It might be that it is possible to discharge one's duties to make the global order more just through benefiting those with whom one transacts. It might also be easier to benefit those with whom one transacts, which could trigger a duty to do so. However, the transaction is unconnected to the grounds for the obligation to repair injustice. Such obligations do not, therefore, seem likely to affect the ethics of transactions against a background of injustice.[8]

Exploitation and how to avoid it

While our duties to repair injustice, arguably, do not depend on the individual transactions in which we are engaged, our duties to avoid exploitation do. According to Alan Wertheimer, one party to a transaction exploits another when she takes *unfair advantage* of him (Wertheimer 1996, 207). Suppose the local water supply is temporarily contaminated and only one, privately owned, well remains. Provided that there are no other sources of clean water, people will pay as much as they can afford for the water, since they need it to survive. If the owner of the well massively increases the price of water, then she will be taking advantage of the local population's need for her water. If we think that it is unfair to charge more for water just because the other supplies are contaminated then she will be taking unfair advantage of the local population, that is, she will be *exploiting* them.

Charges of exploitation are often raised against trans-national transactions. This was the complaint that Indonesia made to justify stopping sharing H5N1 samples – the government thought that they were contributing to a resource whose benefits were going to go to rich countries' citizens, but not to poor Indonesians. When the knowledge of the San people of southern Africa about the appetite-suppressing qualities of *hoodia* was used to develop products for the Western weight loss industry, one of the complaints of the San was that they should have the opportunity to benefit from the commercialization (Wynberg 2004). Their lack of access to the technology needed to commercialize *hoodia* and their open communication about its properties made them vulnerable to exploitation by better resourced and connected outsiders. When it is argued that clinical research in low- and middle-income countries ought to be "responsive" to the health needs of the local populations, the most plausible explanation of why people think this is that they think responsiveness can prevent research from being exploitative (CIOMS 2002, Guideline 10; Millum 2012b).

Social injustice frequently makes exploitation easier. Much of the time, the beneficiaries of injustice have greater bargaining power than the victims of injustice, as a consequence of the disparities between them. Consider, for example, how economic disparities make exploitation more likely. Someone poor is likely to need a given amount of money much more than someone wealthy. She is therefore more likely to agree to terms that are unfair than he is. The wages and working conditions of sweatshops can result from these sorts of disparities. Given sufficient poverty in a population and surplus labour supply, people will agree to work in conditions that are clearly unfair, so long as they are still better off than they would be without the work.[9]

If exploitation occurs when one party takes unfair advantage of another, this suggests two ways in which exploitation can be prevented. The first is to equalize the power disparities between the parties that make it possible for one to take advantage of the other. If two people are roughly economically equal, have access to the same information and so on, then neither will be able to make the other agree to an unfair distribution of benefits. This is one justification, for example, for allowing workers to form unions. The union has greater bargaining power than do individual workers and, normally, in heavily unionized industries it is not easy for an employer to take advantage of a surplus of workers to drive down the wages paid to each.

The other way to prevent exploitation is to ensure that the distribution of the benefits and burdens of the transaction is fair. If the benefits and burdens are distributed fairly, then it is not possible for the more powerful party to take *unfair* advantage of the vulnerable situation of the other.[10] Laws that set minimum wages or that make stipulations about the quality of working conditions can be understood as attempts to prevent unfair agreements about how the benefits and burdens of work are to be distributed.[11] They therefore use this strategy to prevent the exploitation of workers.

Both ways to prevent exploitation face challenges in specifying what is meant by their normative terms. What does it mean for a distribution of benefits and burdens to be fair? There is no agreement on principles of fairness for transactions; rather, much of the time people rely on intuitive judgments (Wertheimer 1996, 207–246). What does it mean for two individuals to have equal power? Neither analytic philosophy nor the bioethics literature provide analyses of power that are easy to apply to the sorts of transactions with which this chapter is concerned.

However, the strategy of preventing exploitation by ensuring that the benefits and burdens of a transaction are fairly distributed has one clear advantage. When there is a difference in power between two parties, trying to equalize their power may be highly problematic. First, it may be very hard to achieve. For example, the privileges of being a Western scientist are not easily given up. Second, quite prudently given the unjust state of the world, people may not want to unilaterally relinquish their power. Third, the mutually beneficial transaction may rely on the advantages of the more powerful party. The Western scientist who renounces her position, ignores funding opportunities and refuses to use her contacts is likely to be of little use to a fellow scientist in an under-resourced institution in sub-Saharan Africa.

By contrast, it is often possible to make the terms of one's transactions fair without running into these problems. The Western scientist can keep her privileges, retain her connections and funding, and yet still work out a memorandum of understanding that ensures that her collaborators are fairly rewarded for their contributions to joint research projects.

Third party beneficiaries

In science and medicine, the majority of the benefits of a project often return to people other than the particular individuals who contribute to it. For example, a disease surveillance programme that takes blood and saliva samples from patients is normally intended to benefit at least the local population, and could be crucial to preventing national or international outbreaks of disease. Likewise, the primary function of medical research is to benefit future patients, not research participants themselves. Indeed, in both of these cases, there are sometimes projects that are not expected to benefit the majority contributors at all, but generate great benefits for other people. The surveillance programme may only have benefits for people who have not already been infected. The research may only result in new clinical interventions years after the participants have died from their disease. How can such projects avoid exploitation?

Notice, first, that the identity of the beneficiaries seems to matter greatly. In the cases I mentioned in the introduction, the complaints of exploitation were levelled at institutions and other actors from rich countries who were perceived as benefiting too much. Part of the grounds for the complaints was that a particular set of people would not benefit – poor Indonesians, patients in LMICs, indigenous populations. But this latter set of people is much larger than the set of people who directly contribute to the project. It was not all Indonesians who were contributing samples to the Global Influenza Surveillance Network. And it is not all members of a host community or nation who participate in a research study. This suggests that exploitation can sometimes be avoided by providing benefits to people who are not themselves parties to the transaction.

Which beneficiaries count? That is, when does a benefit to a third party count towards an assessment of whether the distribution of the burdens and benefits of a transaction is fair? Since the third parties are not themselves involved in the transaction, we must presumably count their interests as in some sense co-extensive with those of a party to the transaction. That party will be contributing to the project *on behalf of* these third parties (and they will, as it were, be benefiting on her behalf). We may distinguish two types of relationships in which this makes sense: *reciprocal relationships* and *relationships of identification*.

Reciprocal relationships occur when people repeatedly interact with each other in ways that provide benefits to both parties. In such cases, while the distribution of benefits and burdens within one transaction may be unequal and not reflect the parties' respective contributions, their transactions taken as a whole may not lead to an unfair distribution of benefits and burdens. For example, within a community, people may work with each other, lend money to each other, share resources, watch each other's children, manage common land, be governed by the same institutions, and so on. One person from the community taking on a burden to help others may reasonably expect reciprocal burdens to be taken on by the others at different times.

Reciprocal relationships need not even require the actual benefits and burdens between parties to balance out. Hypothetical contributions can count here, too, i.e. when one party *would* contribute to a social good or help another, were the occasion to arise. Such hypothetical acts are partly constitutive of some relationships, such as community membership and friendship. Friends not only do, but arguably should, perform favours for one another without accounting. That one person does much more for her friend than he does for her does not imply any unfair treatment, provided that he would do the same for her under the right circumstances. The richer friend regularly pays for dinner, though the poorer one would do so if their circumstances were reversed. Everyone watches the game at the house of the person with the television, though each would host if she were the television owner instead.[12] Only when the opportunity for reciprocation arises and the purported friend fails to do his part is there cause for her to complain that he is not a true friend, or, pertinent to this discussion, that he was exploiting her friendship.

This idea about whose interests count makes sense of why benefits to a person's community or fellow citizens might prevent her from being exploited by an outsider. For example, as noted above, it is commonly thought that research in LMICs that is "responsive", that is, research that addresses an important health problem of the population from which research participants are drawn, is not exploitative. One explanation for this is that the members of the population that benefit are often part of a wider system of reciprocation. Research participants may contribute to the health of others in their community or society. But where others within that population also contribute in different ways, or even where they would contribute if the opportunity arose, the benefits of the research to this population may prevent it from being exploitative.[13]

Relationships of identification occur when someone regards the interests of another as though they were her own. For example, a parent might choose a benefit to her child over a benefit to herself without regarding it as a sacrifice. Spouses and close friends may find that their lives intertwine to the extent that the successes and losses they care about are as much the other person's as their own. In such cases, if the person involved in a transaction reasonably regards the interests in question as equivalent to her own interests, it seems reasonable for others to do so as well. Again, benefits to the other person could then be counted for the avoidance of exploitation.[14]

Reciprocal relationships and relationships of identification frequently coincide. We often interact for mutual benefit with those whom we care about and we naturally come to care about those with whom we beneficially interact. Thus we should expect overlap between these two cases in which benefits to a third party can count towards an assessment of the fairness of the terms of a transaction.

The foregoing analysis of when benefits to a third party can count towards an assessment of the fairness of the terms of a transaction fits well with many people's intuitive judgments about cases. For example, it explains why benefits to the communities from which research participants are drawn can prevent research from being exploitative, even if those communities are not themselves heavily involved in the research. And it correctly places beneficiaries like company shareholders, researchers whose careers are advanced by the research and wealthy patient groups on the other side of the scale. Research may be conducted on behalf of these beneficiaries. But they are not normally the beneficiaries on behalf of whom research participants in LMICs take on burdens and contribute to generalizable knowledge. The benefits to these latter beneficiaries are the ones that must be balanced by benefits to the research participants (or those with whom the research participants have relationships of reciprocation or identification).[15]

Cautionary notes

These conclusions about whose benefits count should be interpreted and implemented with caution. First, we should beware of exacerbating injustice. The fact that people are part of a social system, even one that they endorse, does not entail that their positions with respect to each other are (roughly) fair and thus that it is acceptable to ask one to take on burdens for the sake of another. There is always the risk that the less privileged members of a community will end up bearing burdens from which the more privileged members benefit, or the elite of a country will themselves exploit other members of the population. In general, we should be alert for unjust social structures that make certain people bear burdens for others, and wary of relying on the self-serving testimony of powerful people who claim to speak for others.

Second, whether or not we count a third party's interests depends on whether the person directly involved in the transaction agrees. In these situations, one party to the transaction is asking another to contribute or take on burdens *on behalf of* third parties. It may be that the second party declines to do so. The claim argued for in the previous section is not that the interests of others actually *are* the interests of the person directly involved in the transaction, just that it is acceptable to ask her to count them as such, for the purposes of analysing the transaction's fairness. For example, you cannot unilaterally decide to pay my brother for work I do and thereby claim to have given me a fair deal, even if I identify with his interests. I would have to agree to it.

The other side of this cautionary note is that the contributor's agreement to let certain benefits count is necessary but it is not sufficient for them actually to count for the purposes of assessing a transaction's fairness. With both reciprocal relationships and relationships of identification it is a matter of fact whether the relationship obtains. Whether or not the members of a community are in reciprocal relationships with one another depends on how they do and would help each other. Whether someone identifies with the interests of a distant relative depends on various facts about her relationship to him, her conception of herself and the significance that family has for her. Neither relationship can be created by a simple speech act, such as giving consent.

Conclusions

People are rightly concerned about how to ethically transact with those who are victims of global injustice. I have identified three areas of possible concern: the existence of disparities may encourage the perception of wrongdoing, there may be duties to ameliorate injustice, and disparities between transacting parties make exploitation easier and therefore more likely. Analysis of this last category suggests that it is normally easier to ensure that the benefits and burdens of transactions are shared fairly than to eliminate the power disparities that make it possible for some to take advantage of others. Fair distributions of benefits and burdens can be achieved through the provision of benefits more widely than just to the parties directly involved in a transaction. In particular, it can be helpful to conceptualize the burdens or contributions someone assumes or makes as being on behalf of others. This explains why benefits to community members, fellow disease sufferers or co-nationals can have ethical significance.

Acknowledgements

For helpful comments on earlier drafts of this paper, I would like to thank Erik Malmqvist, Alan Wertheimer, Kristin Zeiler and participants at the *Sharing Bodies within and across Borders* symposium. *Disclaimer*: The views expressed are the author's own. They do not represent the position or policy of the National Institutes of Health, US Public Health Service, or the Department of Health and Human Services. *Funding Support*: This work was supported, in part, by intramural funds from the National Institutes of Health Clinical Center and Fogarty International Center.

Notes

1 Strictly speaking, both parties could be victims of injustice, since I am concerned with any case in which there are significant unjust disparities between the transacting parties. For ease of expression, I continue to describe one as the beneficiary and one as the victim.
2 Compare Rawls (1971, 7).
3 For a brief overview see Millum (2012a, 20–24).
4 The extension to more than two parties should not throw up any additional ethical concerns, though it may generate additional coordination problems.
5 Throughout I describe the party who is more advantaged as the more powerful party. However, this is a simplification. Not only is the concept of power multi-faceted, but the relative power of two individuals is highly sensitive to context. The relative power of a rich tourist in Brazil and a poor slum dweller will change depending on whether the tourist is at his hotel bar or lost in a favela. Likewise, considered as a dyad, a healthy poor person with a kidney to sell may have more power than her rich potential buyer, who urgently needs a transplant. But if there are many people willing to sell their kidneys this power dynamic may reverse. Thanks to Alan Wertheimer for this point.
6 An alternative to the duty to rescue might be something like the second original position posited by Rawls, which he argues leads to a duty on peoples to assist burdened societies (Rawls 1999, 105–113).
7 For an example worked through at greater length see Merritt *et al.* (2010).
8 Similar conclusions have been reached regarding the source of obligations to research participants and host communities. See, e.g., Hughes (2014), and for a contrary view London (2005).

9 I do not mean to imply that all sweatshop labour is freely chosen, only that it can be freely chosen and yet still be exploitative.

10 Article 1 of the Convention on Biological Diversity states: "The objectives of this Convention, to be pursued in accordance with its relevant provisions, are the conservation of biological diversity, the sustainable use of its components and the fair and equitable sharing of the benefits arising out of the utilization of genetic resources" (UN 1992). The requirement for "fair and equitable" benefit-sharing thus writes into the Convention how benefits should be allocated – albeit at a rather abstract level – rather than relying on free, individual negotiations to decide allocations at a case-by-case level.

11 It does not follow that they are successful in doing so – an improvement in the terms of a contract may still not bring the contracting parties to the level of being fairly treated.

12 The rules of friendship are, at least partly, a product of culture. These examples are simply meant to illustrate the existence of conceptions of reciprocal relationships that are familiar from other areas of people's lives.

13 Cf. Millum (2012b) which draws an analogy with how research is (ideally) incorporated into health systems for the benefit of all. Compare the analysis given by Hughes (2012), who argues that it is not justifiable for researchers to ask research participants in LMICs to take on substantial net risks in order to benefit patients in high-income countries. However, he argues that it is permissible to ask such participants to take on substantial net risks to benefit people in their own socio-economic class (or those worse off than they are). Note that Hughes is interested in when it is appropriate to ask people to act altruistically, rather than with how to analyse the fairness of a distribution of benefits.

14 One interesting question concerns how these benefits are to be counted. Someone might, for example, identify much more with the interests of her spouse or child than with her co-nationals. A precise reckoning might analyse this by discounting for more distant relationships. Such precision is outside the bounds of this chapter.

15 There are some interesting grey cases that are illuminated by this analysis. Patients with the same disease may feel solidarity with one another. Such solidarity might constitute an appropriate justification for asking some of them to take on burdens, such as through research participation, for the benefit of others, even if they have no other connection. Similarly, poor populations in different countries might reasonably take on burdens and make contributions on each other's behalves when it would be inappropriate to ask them to do so for more advantaged groups.

References

CIOMS (Council for International Organizations of Medical Sciences). 2002. *International Ethical Guidelines for Biomedical Research Involving Human Subjects.* Geneva: CIOMS/WHO.

Emanuel, E.J. 2008. "Benefits to Host Countries." In: *The Oxford Textbook of Clinical Research Ethics*, edited by E.J. Emanuel, C. Grady, R.A. Crouch, R.K. Lie and F.G. Miller, 719–728. New York: Oxford University Press.

Hughes, R. 2012. "Individual Risk and Community Benefit in International Research." *Journal of Medical Ethics* 38(10): 626–629.

Hughes, R. 2014. "Justifying Community Benefit Requirements in International Research." *Bioethics* 28(8): 397–404.

London, A.J. 2005. "Justice and the Human Development Approach to International Research." *Hastings Center Report* 35(1): 24–37.

Malmqvist, E. 2013. "Taking Advantage of Injustice." *Social Theory and Practice* 39(4): 557–580.

Merritt, M.W., Taylor, H.A., and L.C. Mullany. 2010. "Ancillary Care in Community-based Public Health Intervention Research." *American Journal of Public Health* 100(2): 211–216.

Millum, J. 2010. "How Should the Benefits of Bioprospecting Be Shared?" *Hastings Center Report* 40(1): 24–33.

Millum, J. 2012a. "Global Bioethics and Political Theory." In: *Global Justice and Bioethics*, edited by J. Millum and E.J. Emanuel, 17–42. New York: Oxford University Press.

Millum, J. 2012b. "Sharing the Benefits of Research Fairly: Two Approaches." *Journal of Medical Ethics* 38: 219–223.

Rawls, J. 1971. *A Theory of Justice*. Cambridge, MA and London: Belknap Press of Harvard University Press.

Rawls, J. 1999. *The Law of Peoples*. Cambridge, MA: Harvard University Press.

Sedyaningsih, E.R., Isfandari, S., Soendoro, T., and S.F. Supari. 2008. "Towards Mutual Trust, Transparency and Equity in Virus Sharing Mechanism: The Avian Influenza Case of Indonesia." *Annals, Academy of Medicine, Singapore* 37: 482e8.

Shah, A. 2013. *Poverty Facts and Stats*. Global Issues. www.globalissues.org/article/26/poverty-facts-and-stats.

UN (United Nations). 1992. Convention on Biological Diversity. www.cbd.int/convention/text/default.shtml.

Wertheimer, A. 1996. *Exploitation*. Princeton, NJ: Princeton University Press.

Wynberg, R. 2004. "Rhetoric, Realism and Benefit-Sharing: Use of Traditional Knowledge of Hoodia Species in the Development of an Appetite Suppressant." *Journal of World Intellectual Property* 7(6): 851–876.

13 Concluding reflections

Bodily exchanges as sharing

Erik Malmqvist and Kristin Zeiler

In the introduction to this volume, we described two ethical frameworks that shape much contemporary thinking about bodily exchanges in medicine – the giving and the selling frameworks – and highlighted some of the difficulties that these frameworks face. In this final chapter, we shall tentatively explore an alternative way of framing these exchanges, based on the notion of sharing. In doing so we will draw inspiration from the preceding contributions without, of course, presuming that all contributors will agree with our analysis. We will begin by characterizing the sharing framework, as it might be called, in somewhat greater detail, arguing that it highlights dimensions that the giving and selling frameworks tend to overlook or marginalize. We then examine how the sharing framework fares with respect to common criticisms against these other frameworks and discuss a couple of potential concerns with the notion of sharing. The chapter ends by indicating areas for future inquiry, including some practical issues that might be fruitfully seen through the analytic lens of sharing.

Our aim is not to conclusively establish that the sharing framework is more accurate or ethically appropriate than the giving and selling frameworks, all things considered and across the board.[1] It is entirely possible that the notion of sharing is suitable for some kinds of bodily exchanges in medicine, whereas some other framework is better suited for exchanges of other kinds. It is even possible that the sharing framework raises concerns that are considered weighty enough to undermine its ethical appropriateness in this entire area. These possibilities cannot be assessed without further analysis and debate within and across different scholarly disciplines. Our aim in this chapter is to initiate such analysis and debate.

Outline of a sharing framework

To think of an exchange in terms of sharing is to emphasize its relational or social character. Of course, giving and selling are also relational acts in that they require the involvement of two parties. However, the concept of sharing seems to connote relationality in a more profound sense. First, it is more flexible as regards the number of parties involved in an exchange. The language of giving or selling primarily brings two parties to mind: the giver and the receiver, or the seller and the buyer. Both these parties can certainly be groups of people, and third parties can certainly mediate their exchange. Moreover, what is received or bought can certainly be passed on to another than the original proprietor in a later exchange. Nonetheless, on the most basic level of analysis, the exchange of a gift or commodity is first and foremost a two-party affair. By contrast, the notion of sharing recognizes the *multiple* relationalities that exchanges can involve. Generally speaking, sharing something with someone need not preclude simultaneously sharing it with others as well.

Second, the notion of sharing highlights the *temporally extended* quality that exchanges may have in a way that neither the notion of selling nor that of giving does. To describe an exchange as a sale conveys the idea of a momentaneous event whereby the possession of some good is transferred from one party to another. Once the good and the money have changed hands the deal is over. Gift-giving language is more ambiguous in this regard (Murray 1987). On the one hand, in everyday thought and practice we often assume that giving, like selling, is the momentaneous transfer of a good. On the other hand, we also recognize, as Mauss (1967 [1923–1924]) so forcefully emphasized, that gifts are capable of tying the recipient to the donor over time.[2] The notion of sharing is akin to this latter conception of the gift. It brings to mind, less ambiguously than gift language, the idea of a lasting arrangement that connects the parties over an extended period of time. This difference in temporal emphasis occasionally surfaces in ordinary language. In many cases it makes sense to say that sharing is *continuous* – that we share, for instance, interests or ideals with each other throughout large parts of our lives – whereas corresponding statements dressed in giving (or selling) language would sound odd.

By virtue of these two features, the notion of sharing captures the complex social connections that surround bodily exchanges in medicine more accurately than does either the notion of giving or that of selling. It recognizes that such exchanges can be enabled and shaped by pre-existing relationships and communities, as both de Castro, and Humbracht, Hyun and Lundin highlight in their chapters, or arise from a prior basic sociality, as Zeiler argues in hers. It also recognizes that exchanges in turn can engender new forms of lasting relations, as Sharp, Svenaeus and Toledano discuss in their chapters. This helps make sense of experiences that tend to be puzzling in a giving or selling framework: for instance, the ties that surrogate mothers may feel towards intended parents, and vice versa (see Toledano's chapter); the strongly felt affinities between organ recipients and donors or their kin (see Sharp's chapter); and recipients' uncanny sense of absent donors' presence within (see McCormack's chapter).

The same features also make the notion of sharing a distinct heuristic tool for ethical analysis. Conceptualizing organ and tissue transfer, clinical research and surrogacy in terms of giving or selling tends to encourage a focus on features internal to a temporally isolated two-party exchange. It invites us to ask, for instance, whether either party is harmed in the exchange and whether they engage in it voluntarily. Conceptualizing these practices as a form of sharing broadens the scope of inquiry in two ways. First, in addition to features immediately present in the exchange, this conceptualization encourages examination of the conditions that precede and succeed it, and that may shape and be shaped by it. This invites us to ask whether these conditions are ethically acceptable and whether their acceptability or lack thereof affects the ethics of the exchange itself – questions of the sort that the chapters by Zeiler, McCormack, Malmqvist and Millum broach in different ways.

Second, because it recognizes that parties beyond those immediately involved may have a stake in an exchange, it invites questions about the consequences of the exchange for these parties. Now such questions are quite familiar – the potential effects of different kinds of bodily exchanges on individual third parties, institutions and social practices or norms have received considerable previous attention[3] – and they are by no means impossible to address within a giving or selling framework. Still, they tend to remain somewhat marginalized in these frameworks because of their focus on the two parties immediately involved in the exchange. The sharing framework invites a more inclusive analysis. However, a more systematic identification and scrutiny of third-party effects need not entail giving these effects greater weight. Indeed, the result may even be that undue concerns about such effects are exposed and put to rest. The sharing framework thus paves the way for rigorous ethical analyses of the social and cultural implications of bodily exchanges without legitimizing appealing to such implications in order to set aside the interests of individuals immediately involved.

This broadened inquiry brings questions about distribution and distributive justice to the fore. In a gift-giving framework such questions seem moot. It is improper for the recipient of a gift to complain that the gift was too meagre. And the donor does not have any justice-based claim on the recipient either: reclaiming the gift or demanding a commensurate benefit in return is alien to the ethos of giving (Camenisch 1981; Murray 1987). Similarly, in a selling framework no issue of justice appears to remain once the sale is over. In a paradigmatic market exchange, the fact that a price is voluntarily agreed upon ensures that it is fair.[4] After the deal is done it would be inappropriate for the buyer to demand a partial refund because the price was too high, or for the seller to ask for additional payment because it was too low. In a sharing framework, by contrast, there is potentially an issue of justice that preceeds the exchange and remains after it is over. This is because such a framework recognizes that those involved in and more generally affected by an exchange may be connected by lasting relations and therefore may have responsibilities towards each other that preceed and outlast it (which for recipients need not require giving something of corresponding value back to providers; see below). Indeed, this focus on distributive justice is suggested by the very name of the framework: one meaning of "to share" is to divide benefits as well as burdens between different people. This invites questions about the size of the shares, about who benefits, and about who bears the burdens.

How a sharing framework avoids concerns about giving and selling

As noted in the introduction to this volume, the role of monetary transfers to organ and tissue donors, surrogates and research participants is a perennial concern within the gift framework. This is because money is thought capable of dissolving the act of giving. If I pay for a gift I have received, it is not a genuine gift anymore: its meaning as a gift is displaced or tainted by market valuation (Murray 1987; Campbell 2004). Thus, the gift framework is at pains to distinguish monetary transfers such as reimbursement and compensation, which are considered compatible with giving, from outright purchase, which is thought to turn gifts into commodities – a distinction that has proved difficult to sustain in practice.

In a sharing framework, by contrast, there is no need to draw an artificially sharp distinction in inherently blurred terrain. While payment may annul the gift it does not annul the sharing. There seems to be nothing inconsistent about saying that I share something with someone else and also offering or receiving payment for what is shared. Thus, unlike in the gift framework, the involvement of money is not inherently suspect in a sharing framework. Rather, the appropriateness of money in connection to bodily exchanges in medicine needs to be assessed on a case-by-case basis (cf. Nuffield Council on Bioethics 2011; Hoeyer 2013). Such assessment may lead to the judgment that the involvement of money should be avoided or limited in a particular type of exchange, but the judgment does not precede the assessment.

Thus, using the label "sharing" leaves the question open as to whether it is ethically appropriate that British egg donors are offered subsidized IVF treatment in return for providing eggs for research (see Haimes' chapter) or that Filipino kidney donors receive economic support from recipients (see de Castro's chapter). It may well be that either or both of these arrangements are exploitative or otherwise morally dubious. However, the mere *label* does not settle the issue, as the gift-giving label would.

While the involvement of money is not inherently suspect in a sharing framework, nor is it – unlike in the selling framework – a necessary feature presumed to be in itself unproblematic. The sharing framework is compatible with the view that some kinds of monetary offers in the acquisition of body parts or bodily services are intrinsically wrongful because they amount to treating persons and their bodies as mere objects of market exchange.[5] In other words, it is capable of accommodating the worries about commodification that the selling framework inevitably provokes. Thus, the sharing framework makes it possible to take a nuanced approach to money in relation to bodily exchanges without endorsing a fully fledged market.

One sort of concern with the gift-giving framework is that it hides various potentially troubling aspects of bodily exchanges in medicine (Siminoff and Chillag 1999; Mongoven 2003; Scheper-Hughes 2007). In many cultural settings, gift language evokes images of festive occasions enjoyable to everyone involved, such as birthday or Christmas parties, and of goods offered at relatively low personal expense. Such language may thus trivialize the considerable physical and emotional costs that providers of body parts and bodily services may incur, at least in certain areas of medicine. Moreover, because gifts are by definition voluntarily given (as Bateman emphasizes in her chapter) the fact that providers can be under strong social pressure may be downplayed as well. The language of sharing seems less susceptible to such criticisms. Such language arguably carries fewer overtones of celebration and pleasure than gift language does. It is less likely to suggest that what we talk about is fun or easy. Nor does sharing connote voluntariness to the extent that giving does. A sharing framework thus enables potential concerns that the gift framework glosses over to be acknowledged and analysed.

According to another critique, the gift framework promotes feelings of indebtedness and problematic forms of reciprocation. Empirical research has shown that organ recipients can experience a heavy debt of gratitude towards donors or their kin and a corresponding need to "pay back" what they have received with something of commensurate value (Siminoff and Chillag 1999; Fox and Swazey 2002). Cancelling the debt can, however, be difficult or even impossible when the donor is dead (and so cannot receive reciprocation) and when recipients believe that what they have received is life itself (which is often considered invaluable and cannot be reciprocated in kind). When health professionals frame donation as gift giving they are said to encourage such experiences because they invoke the implicit presumption that gratitude and counter-gifts are precisely what the receipt of a gift requires (Siminoff and Chillag 1999).

Framing the exchange as a form of sharing appears to be less vulnerable to this critique. Of course, transplant recipients may harbour strong and potentially damaging feelings towards donors and their kin in a sharing framework too. But such a framework provides clues about how these feelings may be channelled in more productive directions. A shift from seeing transplant patients as recipients of valuable gifts to seeing them as involved in a sharing relationship entails a corresponding shift in the sort of response that it makes sense for them to engage in. Rather than recognizing the debt by expressing gratitude to donors or their kin or seeking to cancel it by offering counter-gifts, an appropriate response may be to affirm the connections that transplantation engenders. This could mean, for instance, embracing the sort of relational work Sharp describes in her contribution to this volume. Another response may be to expand such connections further by sharing one's body with yet others in need, for instance through oneself registering as a potential post-mortem donor. Thus, a sharing framework is capable of acknowledging the urge to respond to the receipt of an organ without promoting "the tyranny of the gift" that Fox and Swazey (2002, 40) identified (cf. Zeiler 2014b).

Unease about sharing

While a framework of sharing avoids certain difficulties with the giving and selling frameworks, it also raises potential concerns that need to be addressed.

Two concerns stand out in particular. First, conceptualizing bodily exchanges as sharing might be taken to imply that people's bodies are not really theirs but rather belong to the larger community. The implication, in other words, is that a person's body is a shared resource that may be used for the common good with little or no regard for the person's own wishes. Second, contrary to our suggestion that the language of sharing invites a focus on distributive justice, it might be argued that such language actually conceals or even promotes unjust inequalities. Speaking of sharing may create the impression that everyone is involved on equal terms. This may fail to recognize that some take an unduly large portion of shared benefits or assume an unduly small portion of shared burdens – and even perhaps encourage such conduct.

These concerns are to be taken seriously, but we believe that they can be accommodated by suitable amendments and qualifications. A sharing framework surely cannot be expected to do all the analytic work alone. If it is to yield adequate ethical analyses of bodily exchanges in medicine it needs to be coupled with additional, independent ethical considerations. In this respect a sharing framework is no different from the giving or selling frameworks.

Thus, in response to the first concern, we do not suggest that adopting a sharing framework would involve abandoning consent as a necessary condition for most bodily exchanges in medicine. Using people's bodies in ways to which they have not voluntarily agreed would generally be proscribed, as is presumably the case in a giving or selling framework. To be sure, there are genuine questions as to what counts as valid consent and when consent is required. Does presumed consent to post-mortem organ donation qualify as consent in a morally robust sense? Is re-consent needed for using tissue samples for other research projects than those for which the samples were first procured? But these are independent questions about the meaning and role of consent: they arise no matter which framework one adopts.

Still, it might be argued that framing bodily exchanges as sharing could create expectations that people share their bodies with others when they would rather not. In other words, the sharing framework might engender or reinforce social pressure on individuals to donate organs, tissues or cells, agree to surrogacy arrangements or participate in clinical research. This is a legitimate worry, and anyone who uses the language of sharing to name or promote these practices in real-world healthcare settings should be wary of such effects. That said, remember that concerns about social pressure arise, in different ways, in a giving or selling framework as well (Scheper-Hughes 2007; Malmqvist 2014). Indeed, given the high stakes, there will arguably always be a risk that people are pressured to engage in these practices – regardless of how they are conceptualized. Thus, there is arguably a need to detect and minimize such pressures under any ethical framework.

In response to the second concern, it should be stressed that when talking about sharing one must not forget to ask who is included among those who share, and how large are the benefits they enjoy and the burdens they bear. As we noted above, the sharing framework brings such questions into view, which is a clear advantage if one wants to detect and analyse any distributive inequities that bodily exchanges may involve. But the framework does not itself incorporate any particular conception of distributive justice, and so it must be combined with some such conception for the analysis to be complete.

Nonetheless, there may be reason for concern about sharing as a rhetorical device rather than an analytic tool. Perhaps sharing language is useful for powerful parties who wish to silence justice-based claims from the less powerful: “You too get a share, so don’t complain”. Again, any enterprise that publicly names or promotes bodily exchanges as sharing should be cautious of such abuses. However, it is unclear that a sharing rhetoric is more problematic in this regard than, say, a giving or selling rhetoric. Gift language seems to enable the better off to encourage the worse off to provide body parts and bodily services without expecting anything in return, and market language enables them to claim that a voluntarily accepted sum of money is adequate reciprocation. Sharing language, by contrast, appears to enable the worse off to insist that access to their bodies is not unconditional. It also enables them to demand other things than money in return – for instance, adequate insurance or post-trial access to treatments in the case of clinical research. There is, then, arguably something potentially empowering about sharing language.

Looking forward

In this chapter we have examined the notion of sharing as a possible starting point for ethical analyses of bodily exchanges in medicine. We have outlined the main elements of a sharing framework, distinguishing it from the giving and selling frameworks that shape much previous ethical debate in this area. We have argued that the sharing framework has some distinct advantages over these other frameworks, but also raised a couple of concerns that require attention. Our discussion has proceeded on a rather general level, with relatively little attention to concrete issues of practical concern. Yet part of the attractiveness of a sharing framework hinges on its ability to inspire compelling analyses of such issues. While any comprehensive analyses of this sort must wait, we will nonetheless end this chapter by indicating a few concrete ethical issues where this framework may prove illuminating.

Two such issues have been touched upon already but can be pursued a little further. The first one concerns how organ donation should be described in the clinical as well as the public setting. Our suggestion that sharing language is less likely than giving language to hide the downsides of transplantation and reinforce damaging indebtedness among recipients has implications both for the dialogue between professionals and patients and for public campaigns aimed at encouraging donation. To be sure, accurate and transparent communication is a delicate and complex task in both these areas, and any choice of language will have practical implications that require continuous critical attention (cf. Siminoff and Chillag 1999). Nonetheless, our analysis tentatively supports incorporating the notion of sharing in this communication and encourages inquiries into how that might be accomplished in practice.[6]

The second issue we have already broached is the involvement of money in bodily exchanges. In keeping with the Nuffield Council on Bioethics' (2011) recent analysis, the sharing framework takes a nuanced and contextual approach to this issue. The appropriateness of financial transfers to providers of body parts and bodily services is to be assessed on a case-by-case basis, without trying to determine whether any particular transfer is consistent with gift-giving or instead amounts to a purchase. This makes the framework a promising starting point for examining and problematizing exchanges where money is involved in ways that tend to escape or collapse these familiar categories, including "egg sharing" for treatment and research (see Haimes' chapter) and payment of funeral expenses for deceased organ donors (Delmonico *et al.* 2002). For the same reason, the framework enables transparent analyses of practices where money is ostensibly offered as reimbursement or compensation but de facto functions as a financial incentive, as may be the case in reproductive donation (Cooper and Waldby 2014) and clinical research (Elliott and Abadie 2008). To repeat, it is entirely possible that the involvement of money should be avoided or limited in some or all of these cases. However, this can only be determined on the basis of a careful and contextually attuned analysis.

These two issues aside, the sharing framework seems useful for examining different kinds of *reciprocal* arrangements in regard to bodily exchanges. In such arrangements, those who provide body parts or bodily services contribute on the condition that they, or someone they care about, will benefit in return (unlike in a gift exchange). However, these benefits take a non-monetary form (unlike in a market exchange). In the realm of kidney donation, this happens in cases of "cross-donation" or "kidney exchange" (Roth *et al.* 2004; see also Sharp's chapter). In these cases, a donor who is incompatible with her own designated recipient instead donates to an unknown recipient; in return, the donor's recipient gets a kidney from another donor/recipient pair in a similar situation or is afforded priority in the queue for cadaver kidneys. A similar setup has been proposed for reproductive donation: couples in need of donor eggs would receive reduced waiting time if they provide sperm for another couple in need of sperm donation, and vice versa (Pennings 2007).

On the face of it, the sharing framework appears generally supportive of such arrangements. Its emphasis on distributive justice clearly resonates with the idea that those who take on burdens to help others also benefit in return. On the other hand, the sharing framework also brings critical questions into view. It encourages us to look beyond the parties immediately involved in such arrangements and ask who might be excluded from or disadvantaged by them and whether such exclusion or disadvantaging is justifiable. Is it reasonable, for instance, that single reproducers in need of donor gametes cannot cut their waiting time by contributing to a reciprocal system (Krolokke 2014)? The sharing framework also invites questions about the conditions from which such arrangements arise. Is there a risk, for instance, that people agree to participate because they have been unduly pressured by close ones who are eager for a transplant or a child (Pennings 2007)?

The notion of sharing might invite thinking about reciprocity in broader terms, beyond two-party exchanges. As has been repeatedly illustrated in this volume, it is not uncommon that people contribute body parts and bodily services to large-scale collective enterprises or exchange systems that benefit many, but from which they themselves do not stand to gain, or stand to gain much less than others. Participants in international clinical trials may help develop beneficial drugs that they and others in their communities will be unable to afford. Patients may provide tissue samples that contribute to the growth of knowledge and financial capital without enjoying a share of these goods. People with limited access to healthcare systems wherein organs are distributed may be asked to donate post mortem. Many similar examples come to mind. Any systematic critical appraisal of such wide, non-reciprocal forms of circulation, and any cogent proposal for more reciprocal arrangements, would require a substantive conception of distributive justice that we have not defended here. Yet, the notion of sharing, as we have developed it, appears to point in the direction of this sort of inquiry.

Notes

1 While we do not here aim to exclude the possibility that a giving or selling framework may be the preferable approach to any particular kind of bodily exchange, we have elsewhere questioned the appropriateness of a selling framework in the organ transplantation context (Malmqvist 2014, 2015) and problematized the property rights discourse that tends to underpin such frameworks more generally (Zeiler 2014a).

2 Whereas the Maussian conception of the gift has greatly influenced critical scholarship on bodily exchanges in medicine, it is arguably the other conception that primarily informs the gift-giving framework, understood as a normative framework that specifies how such exchanges ought to be performed and regulated. It is, for instance, this conception of gifts as momentaneous and "free" that transplant professionals invoke to discourage communication between families of deceased donors and organ recipients (see Sharp's chapter). This also appears to be the underlying idea when gift language is used to condemn payment in policy statements. When we contrast sharing with giving throughout this chapter, it is therefore this non-Maussian conception of the gift that we have in mind. We recognize that a revised giving framework, which instead builds on the Maussian conception, might be able to do much of the analytic work that we argue that the sharing framework enables (see Bateman's chapter). However, rather than revising the giving framework we provide a distinct one, avoiding altogether the notion of the gift. In our view, this is a less ambiguous way of recognizing the extended temporalities and social connections that surround bodily exchanges. It also appears less vulnerable to concerns about indebtedness and problematic counter-gifts (see below).

3 For instance, one worry about paid bodily exchanges in the reproductive realm is that they might change the social meaning of parenthood and family relationships (Murray 1996). Similarly, the potential effects of payment for bodily material on societal values like solidarity and altruism have been debated ever since Titmuss'

(1970) classic work on blood donation (Nuffield Council on Bioethics 2011). Though less prominent in debates about clinical research, concerns about social effects sometimes surface there too, for instance in discussions about whether the public might lose trust in the entire research enterprise if they perceive that particular trials are conducted in unethical ways (Malmqvist *et al.* 2011).

4 In other words, justice in market exchange tends to be assessed in accordance with the first part of the dual libertarian thesis that any distribution, however unequal, is just if it results from (i) voluntary transfer of holdings that (ii) were themselves justly acquired (Nozick 1974).

5 The sharing framework outlined here does not presuppose, but is only compatible with, the view that some kinds of monetary offers are intrinsically wrongful because they involve treating people's bodies as mere objects of market exchange. While the framework could certainly be combined with that view, this would require independent argument. It is crucial to note that this by no means precludes forceful critique of a market approach to the body. Indeed, we have developed such a critique elsewhere (Malmqvist 2014, 2015; Zeiler 2014a). The point is merely that such a critique requires independent ethical tools that are not part of the sharing framework as such. For an understanding of the notion of sharing that contrasts more strongly with selling than the one presented here, see Zeiler (2014b).

6 Over fifteen years ago Siminoff and Chillag (1999, 41) noted that the donation-promoting slogan "Share your life, share your decision" was gaining recognition, and cited this slogan as a promising alternative to the "gift of life" discourse that they identified as both deeply entrenched and ethically problematic (cf. Mongoven 2003). However, it seems that the gift remains the "sanctioned metaphor" (Gunnarsson and Svenaeus 2012, 12) in this context, and that sharing language remains comparatively rarely used.

References

Camenisch, P.F. 1981. "Gift and Gratitude in Ethics." *Journal of Religious Ethics* 9: 1–34.

Campbell, C.S. 2004. "The Gift and the Market: Cultural and Symbolic Perspectives." In: *Transplanting Human Tissue: Ethics, Policy, and Practice*, edited by S.J. Youngner, M.W. Anderson and R. Schapiro, 139–159. Oxford: Oxford University Press.

Cooper, M., and C. Waldby. 2014. *Clinical Labor: Tissue Donors and Research Subjects in the Global Bioeconomy.* Durham: Duke University Press.

Delmonico, F.L., Arnold, R., Scheper-Hughes, N., Siminoff, L.A., Kahn, J., and S.J. Youngner. 2002. "Ethical Incentives – Not Payment – for Organ Donation." *New England Journal of Medicine* 346: 2002–2005.

Elliott, C., and R. Abadie. 2008. "Exploiting a Research Underclass in Phase 1 Clinical Trials." *New England Journal of Medicine* 358: 2316–2317.

Fox, R., and J. Swazey. 2002. *Spare Parts: Organ Replacement in American Society.* New York: Oxford University Press.

Gunnarsson, M., and F. Svenaeus. 2012. "Introduction." In: *The Body as Gift, Resource, and Commodity: Exchanging Organs, Tissues, and Cells in the 21st Century*, edited by M. Gunnarsson and F. Svenaeus, 9–30. Huddinge: Södertörn Studies in Practical Knowledge.

Hoeyer, K. 2013. *Exchanging Human Bodily Material: Rethinking Bodies and Markets.* Dordrecht: Springer.

Krolokke, C. 2014. "Eggs and Euros: A Feminist Perspective on Reproductive Travel from Denmark to Spain." *International Journal of Feminist Approaches to Bioethics* 7(2): 144–163.

Malmqvist, E. 2014. "Are Bans on Kidney Sales Unjustifiably Paternalistic?" *Bioethics* 28: 110–118.

Malmqvist, E. 2015. "Kidney Sales and the Analogy with Dangerous Employment." *Health Care Analysis* 23: 107–121.

Malmqvist, E., Juth, N., Lynöe, N., and G. Helgesson. 2011. "Early Stopping of Clinical Trials: Charting the Ethical Terrain." *Kennedy Institute of Ethics Journal* 21: 51–78.

Mauss, M. 1967 [1923–1924]. *The Gift: Forms and Functions of Exchange in Archaic Societies.* Translated by I. Cunnison. New York: Norton.

Mongoven, A. 2003. "Sharing Our Body and Blood: Organ Donation and Feminist Critiques of Sacrifice." *Journal of Medicine and Philosophy* 28: 89–114.

Murray, T.H. 1987. "Gifts of the Body and the Needs of Strangers." *Hastings Center Report* 17(2): 30–38.

Murray, T.H. 1996. *The Worth of a Child.* Berkeley: University of California Press.

Nozick, R. 1974. *Anarchy, State, and Utopia.* Oxford: Blackwell.

Nuffield Council on Bioethics. 2011. *Human Bodies: Donation for Medicine and Research.* London: Nuffield Council on Bioethics.

Pennings, G. 2007. "Mirror Gametes Donation." *Journal of Psychosomatic Obstetrics & Gynecology* 28: 187–191.

Roth, A.E., Sönmez, T., and M. Utku Ünver. 2004. "Kidney Exchange." *Quarterly Journal of Economics* 119: 457–488.

Scheper-Hughes, N. 2007. "The Tyranny of the Gift: Sacrificial Violence in Living Donor Transplants." *American Journal of Transplantation* 7: 507–511.

Siminoff, L.A. and K. Chillag. 1999. "The Fallacy of the 'Gift of Life'." *Hastings Center Report* 29(6): 34–41.

Titmuss, R.M. 1970. *The Gift Relationship: From Human Blood to Social Policy.* London: Allen and Unwin.

Zeiler, K. 2014a. "Neither Property Right Nor Heroic Gift, Neither Sacrifice Nor Aporia – The Benefit of the Theoretical Lens of Sharing in Donation Ethics." *Medicine, Health Care and Philosophy* 17: 171–181.

Zeiler, K. 2014b. "A Phenomenological Approach to the Ethics of Transplantation Medicine: Sociality and Sharing when Living-with and Dying-with Others." *Theoretical Medicine and Bioethics* 35: 369–388.

Index